"In my thirty years as a yoga practitioner, this is one of the few books that has captured the essence of the original holistic meaning and practice of Yoga in a beautiful down-to-earth manner."
—Gabriel Cousens, M.D., MD (H), Diplomat in Ayurveda, Tree of Life Foundation, www.treeoflife.nu, author of *Conscious Eating*.

MASTERING THE SECRETS OF YOGA FLOW

*A Unique Program to Improve Focus, Achieve Peace,
and Reach Full Physical and Mental Potential*

Doug Swenson

A PERIGEE BOOK

A Perigee Book
Published by The Berkley Publishing Group
A division of Penguin Group (USA) Inc.
375 Hudson Street
New York, New York 10014

Perigee trade paperback edition / January 2004

ISBN: 0-399-52945-4

Visit our website at
www.penguin.com

LIBRARY OF CONGRESS CATALOGING-IN-PUBLICATION DATA

Swenson, Doug.
    Mastering the secrets of yoga flow : Sadhana / Doug Swenson.—1st Perigee ed.
    p. cm.
    ISBN 0-399-52945-4
    1. Yoga. 2. Sådhana. I. Title: Sadhana. II. Title.

RA781.7.S947 2004
613.7'046—dc22

2003062906

Printed in the United States of America

10 9 8 7 6 5 4 3 2 1

I would like to dedicate this book to Patanjali, author of the first known book on Yoga, dated 400 B.C. If it were not for Patanjali's great efforts in documenting the practice of yoga, very little information would be available for us today. I would also like to dedicate this book to the ultimate best within each and every one of you and hope this book will touch your heart and mind, inspiring your kindness, compassion, and creativity.

ACKNOWLEDGMENTS

The following people were extremely helpful in putting this project together. My thanks and appreciation goes out to:

Pamela Liflander—Thank you, Pamela, for your many suggestions, talent, and assistance with writing this book. Thank you for your wonderful editing.

Carol Mann—Thank you, Carol, for your suggestions, effort, and assistance with the manuscript and in locating a wonderful publisher.

Sheila Curry Oakes—Special thanks to Sheila Curry Oakes for your faith and support in publishing this book.

Ram Photography—Thank you very much for your great work in producing these fantastic photographs.

Anna Ferguson—Thank you, Anna, for your energy and compassion, and all your assistance in the details of creating the book, including shooting the cover photograph.

Violet Swenson—Thanks, Mother, for all your help with mailing packages and assisting with e-mail.

Mother Nature, Universal Goddess—A very special thanks to Mother Nature for being there when I needed you most and for providing me with the incentive and energy to finish this work.

CONTENTS

INTRODUCTION

I first started practicing yoga some thirty-two years ago. For years I concentrated on mastering the postures, just like everyone else. Then one day I was practicing yoga outdoors and happened to notice my shadow cast across the grass. I began playing with my shadow, watching it change as I entered and exited my yoga postures. As I watched my movements, I became very aware of the picture I was creating: my movements looked very soft and graceful. The flowing motions looked really magical as my shadow danced on the grass.

At the same time I felt something new inside of me. The feeling from my yoga practice when I flowed from one posture to the next was absolutely wonderful.

From that moment on I tried to re-create that incredible feeling. First I thought it was the sequence of postures. Then I realized it was the unique flow from one posture to the next that created this euphoric feeling. The more I practiced outdoors, the more I was able to re-create that energy. When I wasn't doing yoga, I found myself watching the way the flowers danced in the wind, how the clouds floated effortlessly like dreams, and how the rivers displayed both softness and strength. In time I became very in tune to which movements worked best with which postures. Without knowing it, I was creating energy-compatible links, or *vinyasa*.

As I gradually became comfortable with my practice, I realized my whole life was changing for the better. I was nicer to my parents, I could communicate better with all my friends, I found my job less stressful, my surfing improved greatly, I had a desire to eat healthy food, and I actually loved my yoga practice. My mind was feeling quite open and I found myself wanting to learn more about life. My diet was expanding toward a cleaner vegan existence; I would climb a high plateau in the desert at sunset, just to feel the energy of doing yoga on nature's stage.

My yoga is now a reflection of the softness, strength, and energy of nature. My connecting links flow in sync with the same energy, which governs the flow of the whole universe. Circular energy flows returning to the beginning and going with the natural flow of energy, rather than fighting against it.

I have created Sadhana Yoga as more than just a way to practice yoga. It is a wonderful path to living to your full potential and loving every moment of it. After searching many years for answers in churches and in temples, contemplating answers from Earth and in Heavens, I found that all along the answers were very close at hand; they were within my own true self.

Yoga Today

Yoga has never been more popular. From aging baby boomers with aches and pains to a younger, fitter audience, the appeal of yoga is universal. Yoga requires almost no equipment and can be done anywhere, alone or in a group. Its healing properties help strengthen all of the muscles of the body through systematic resistance. It can help you lose weight, release stress, detoxify your body, gain flexibility, increase circulation, and raise your metabolism. Yoga can also help to achieve better concentration and mental focus.

Thirty years ago there were only a few styles of yoga to choose from. Now there are many varieties of yoga, each appealing to different types of people. Some people are drawn to the various hard styles of *Hatha* Yoga, which are based on the yoga postures: powerful movements of the body with less emphasis on inner peace, deep relaxation, and the release of stress and tension. Others are intrigued by softer styles of *Hatha* Yoga, which are the less physical styles that focus on gentle movements and relaxation, or *Raja* Yoga, which embraces the mastery of the mind and a path to enlightenment. All forms of yoga are very beneficial, and I respect each of the different styles and feel they are doing a great service for the whole world. At the same time I feel there is no one style, or *guru*, with all the answers.

Imagine if you could practice a holistic style of yoga which encompassed both enormous strength, blissful relaxation, and spirituality and embraced a continuous flow of energy which could touch your whole life in a positive way, navigating a sacred path through the universe. Today, such a system does exist. The system I speak of is a completely new holistic approach to yoga practice. Combining the feeling of continuous motion, such as found in tai chi with traditional yoga postures, breathing techniques, and enhanced diet, I have created a holistic approach to yoga that connects the vital life force energy of exercise with the spiritual flow of the universe. After your very first experience of practicing with this style you will find your body and mind greatly enhanced, leaving you with a euphoric feeling which can last for hours.

I refer to this new style as Sadhana Yoga, which translates as meaning "practice quest, or act of mastery." Through Sadhana Yoga we strive to embrace a purity of energy, allowing yoga practice to become a true vision of the heart. By moving our energy in circular patterns, we become synchronized with the natural world. Through my unique system you will enjoy the many health benefits of traditional yoga practices, and much, much more.

Sadhana Yoga has a positive, uplifting effect on your mind, creating more mental clarity and focus. Once you find yourself connected with the energy flow in yoga practice, it becomes easy to connect yourself more completely to other aspects of your life. For example, you will gain the confidence and willpower to improve your diet, achieve more productive work, experience stronger personal relationships, enjoy better sleep, and develop a deep passion for life.

Done properly, Sadhana Yoga is an elegant moving meditation, an internal flow with external effects. If you can achieve harmony and grace within your yoga routine, this same energy is carried into your daily world with unlimited positive effects.

I have developed the Sadhana Yoga program over the past thirty years. The inspiration for this method has evolved from having a connection with nature, studying various styles of yoga, and at the same time practicing both a healthy diet and a positive outlook on life. As a result, my daily life incorporates a holistic view which is constantly moving with the flow of yoga and all living things. To me, Sadhana Yoga is more than just a yoga system: it is a way of life.

My system of yoga is based on the teachings of Patanjali, the author of the "Yoga Sutras," who was the first to gather and record the details of the yoga oral tradition in 400 B.C. The masters of this philosophy documented a path to self-enlightenment by connecting the body with *prana*, the universal energy flow. The techniques were based on the supremacy of the natural world. Through yoga, one was able to harness the natural energy flow, which then would physically and mentally enhance one's life.

A New Approach to Flow and Yoga

Within the many styles of yoga, the word *flow* has certainly been used before, such as in "Flow Yoga," or "*Vinyasa* Flow." In these instances and in most others, the word *flow* refers to creating a generic connecting link between postures. In some cases, the word *flow* has very little to do with any movements of the body within yoga practice. In other cases, yoga teachers might practice *Vinyasa* Flow with some fluid movements, but do not have an overall holistic approach, so their yoga practice is often taught without proper sequencing and a scattered energy flow. Other styles of yoga that incorporate generic connecting links cater mostly to the very fit student, such as *Ashtanga* or Power Yoga.

My system links the traditional yoga postures in a proper sequence with new and unique flowing transitional movements. I've also created a few base *vinyasa*, for training energy lines. These transitions allow the energy produced through the proper completion of each posture to continue flowing. The additional transitional movements, coupled with specific yoga breathing, create a beautiful, flowing line of energy between yoga postures. My flowing links can be added between any yoga posture, in any style of practice. By embracing the fundamentals of Sadhana Yoga, you can greatly improve all styles of yoga practice.

The flow of Sadhana Yoga is holistic; it is all about the natural flow of energy in life and how we can reconnect with this energy through yoga practice, diet, and lifestyle. In Sadhana Yoga we incorporate the complete ideal of yoga practice, catering to all ages, shapes and sizes. Sadhana Yoga can at the same time be more physical than other styles, or softer than a quiet walk in the park. The choice is up to you!

STRUCTURE OF THE BOOK

Sadhana Yoga is recommended for beginners and accomplished students alike, coupled with easy-to-follow instructions on how to create the flowing links for each posture. By reading this book, you will gain an increased understanding of the existing yoga styles, and see why Sadhana Yoga is so vastly different. You'll quickly learn how to introduce its lessons into your yoga practice and adopt a whole new way of life.

There is a complete listing of all of the yoga postures and flowing links, featuring detailed descriptions and photographs that show how to complete the postures, and information on all of their various benefits, including workouts for beginners through advanced with a variety of routines to suite your needs.

Finally, you will learn about the teachings of Sadhana Yoga beyond your mat, with many suggestions on how to greatly enhance your life. This section includes complete information on the many positive benefits of getting regular exercise, understanding the practices of relaxation and meditation, and learning how to fuel your body properly for increased energy. Lastly, you will come to understand the philosophical teachings of Sadhana Yoga so that you can recognize your life's true purpose.

If you can experience this gift as I have, you will quickly see how the benefits of Sadhana Yoga are endless.

Namaste,
Doug
August 2003

PART I

DISCOVERING

SADHANA YOGA

FLOW

GETTING IN TOUCH WITH YOUR NATURAL FLOW

Embrace the energy

The natural flow of life

will become you

The most central idea to any yoga practice and particularly to Sadhana Yoga is *prana*, which means "vital life force." The vital life force refers to the spark that separates living beings from nonliving material. It is the core within which connects all of us to the universe. In today's often hectic world many of us have become very disconnected from nature and its flow of energy. We tend to fight against nature and the laws of nature rather than going with the flow. Through yoga, and specifically through Sadhana Yoga, we can return to, and connect with, the natural current of the vital life force. This means gaining greater inner peace and a strong sense of physical well-being.

The vital life force is not unique to people. From the smallest single-cell animal to the infinite energy of a million galaxies and everything in between, the entire natural world is connected through the energy found in all organisms. Each of us can learn to harness this natural energy and reap the benefits of living closer to the vital life force. From this vibrant current we can fuel our lives. It drives us to reach our personal best no matter what we choose to do. Just as a fish separated from water cannot live, and the beautiful colors of a flower cannot be seen without light, humans cannot reach their full potential if they live apart from the natural flow of universal energy.

Of course, people achieve varying degrees of the vital life force: it is not simply an "all or nothing" concept. If you are alive, then you are embracing some degree of *prana*. However, some people have a very weak vital life current, while others experience one that is very strong. The effects can mean the difference between living a full, active, and healthy life, to simply going through the motions. Those who embrace *prana* can be completely focused, at peace, and reach their full potential both physically and mentally. However, if you choose to remove yourself from the natural flow and drift away from nature, the connection is broken and the vital life force within you cannot grow.

Connecting with Prana: The Power of the Elements

All plants, insects, animals, and microorganisms live by the laws of nature. All life is energy: it is only manifested in different forms. This *prana* energy is transferred to all life forms through the five elements: Earth, air, fire, water, and ether. The five elements are the conduits that sustain us and deliver the vital life force to our own bodies.

The **Earth** is much more than a round rock hurtling through space. Earth is alive, full of energy and the vital life force. Just as you have veins with warm blood pulsing throughout your body and into your heart, our planet Earth has rivers of warm molten lava traveling throughout its vast extremities and into its heart. Just as you have lungs to breathe and to filter pollution, the Earth has trees and plants to do this work.

The Earth is a part of you and you are a part of the Earth. If you disrespect the Earth through waste and pollution, in essence you are destroying a part of yourself as well. Within the spectrum of Sadhana Yoga you will learn to move in sync with the rhythm and energy of the Earth by awakening your full potential through a unique combination of breathing techniques, yoga postures, connecting links, and high-quality diet. In time you will become in tune with the natural rhythm of the Earth, be more grounded in your yoga practice, and mentally be true to your convictions even when you are surrounded by opposition.

The element **Air** translates for our use as oxygen, and to us this means life. There is a wonderful buddy system whereby we inhale oxygen and exhale carbon dioxide, and in exchange plants exhale oxygen and inhale carbon dioxide. The amount and quality of oxygen you consume dictates a large part of your prana energy level.

In Sadhana Yoga you will be asked to take slow, deep, and complete inhalations and exhalations, in order to fully utilize all the benefits of air within your yoga practice. In time you will learn to use synchronized breathing techniques and ride your breath, much like a surfer on a wave, creating a very strong flowing practice. By enhancing your breathing techniques, you will find a very sacred connection with all life and feel more in touch with nature and the Earth itself. Your mind will feel clear, and your friends will find your presence exhilarating; a literal breath of fresh air.

The element of **Fire** can be translated as meaning heat. Without heat we would all freeze. Without the sun nothing could grow and all life as we know it would cease. In the yogic tradition we are taught to salute the sun's life-giving warmth and energy at sunrise and sunset. Scientifically we know that moderate sun exposure can greatly enhance your health and mental state. This moderate sunlight can enhance your immune system, release tension, help detoxify your body, and pull you closer to the natural rhythm of the universe.

Beyond the physical heat from the sun, Sadhana Yoga will teach you to create heat within your own body. The vision of internal core heat from your yoga practice will keep your body warm, and the light of higher consciousness from all aspects of your yoga and diet will radiate to all those around you, much like the sun itself.

Water is another magical element with which we cannot do without. Water comes in three forms: liquid, ice, and vapor. You can use water for exterior cleansing, interior cleansing, hydrating your body, and for the soothing and tranquil effects of swimming. You can learn much from watching the softness and strength of a river as it makes its way through the countryside: it is beautiful yet powerful enough to cut through rock.

Sadhana Yoga will teach you that like water, you can be both soft and powerful as your yoga practice flows with grace. This same energy of fluid softness will help you in everyday life, as you learn to be free flowing, yet very powerful in communication.

Ether is the word used to describe the voids of deep space beyond our atmosphere. It was once thought to be an invisible elastic substance filling the space between distant objects. Later studies suggested that ether is nothing at all, just a void of substance, or a vacuum. Gravity, light, and energy pass through this void of nothingness to bring us life.

Ether is then the medium which allows invisible energy to pass through its space as a connecting link to distant shores.

Our bodies are also mediums that carry energy. Through the practice of Sadhana Yoga you can learn a lesson from ether. There are times when it is good to be nothing, void of all, calm and quiet as you let the energy of life pass through you. At other times your yoga practice will allow your body to connect to the Earth in order to receive the vital life force. Whether you are active or perfectly still, you can control how the energy of life comes to you.

The Power of Nature

Long before I was a yogi I embraced the oceans as a surfer. I held the philosophy that to master the oceans I had to master its energy. Once I was surfing in Hawaii and almost drowned when I went against the flow of energy, as a huge wave pounded me under tons of ocean water. I woke up on the beach shaking, and I gazed back at the softness and beauty of the powerful waves folding gracefully on the offshore reef. I then realized you could never master the power of nature: if you want to succeed, you have to go with the natural flow, and have the power and energy of nature working with you, not against you.

The goal of Sadhana Yoga is to both release and harness the subtle energy flow within all of us and connect it naturally to the greater external flow of nature. Through this connection in our yoga practice we can achieve a deepening inner peace and greater harmony in our lives.

The Movement of the Universe

The universe is quite vast and mind-boggling, yet at the same time very simplistic. Most of us think of the universe in terms of the larger energy forms such as stars and galaxies. Yet just as important are the smaller aspects of the universe, such as molecules and atoms, which in turn make up the larger celestial bodies.

There is at least one common thread running throughout the whole universe: all things are moving in a circular motion. Planets and their moons orbit the roundness of the sun. Galaxies are formed and spin around much like the clouds of a hurricane photographed from above. And on the smallest scale, inside an atom you will find electrons, protons and neutrons, all spinning around like miniature solar systems.

The philosophy of yoga is to become connected with the universe and the natural flow of life. Sadhana Yoga has evolved from this ancient practice to create a very circular form of movement, replicating the energy patterns of the universe both large and small.

All Energy Becomes One

We now understand that all of our interactions with the elements are a form of energy. You can then divide this energy into two categories: the visually witnessed energy and invisible energy. Examples of energy you can see are waves crashing on the beach, tree roots that have grown through a rock, a plant reaching toward the sun, or a lightning bolt flashing out of the sky. Examples of invisible energy are gravity, sound passing through ether, and the energy of the vital life force. When you practice Sadhana Yoga, you will learn to become a part of both the visible and the invisible energy. When you tie it all together, your practice becomes one with the energy of the whole universe.

ENHANCING YOUR VITAL LIFE FORCE

The primary catalyst for enhancing your vital life force is through my special technique of Sadhana Yoga practice, which links traditional yoga postures together through the creation of unique flowing movements. These flowing movements increase the energy flow and reconnect you to the vital life force. While yoga practice allows you to create the *prana* energy of the vital life force, if you practice each yoga posture separately, this energy becomes somewhat dissipated. To derive the maximum energy from your yoga practice, you need to connect the postures together with a flowing energy link. The flowing links in Sadhana Yoga are called *vinyasa* and serve as an invisible wire connecting the energy from one posture to the next, just as power lines connect electricity from one house to the main electrical plant.

My style of practice will teach you how to continually move the energy lines of each individual pose. This unique technique of Sadhana Yoga is considered by many to be the most beautiful style of yoga practice: simultaneously creating harmony within, while outwardly exhibiting a graceful strength.

Building Your Body

The body itself is an amazing, natural machine that must be in motion on a regular basis or it will break down. Paul Bragg, a famous health advocate and world-renowned healer, once said; "To rest is to rust." When it comes to improving the shape and condition of your body, all fitness professionals will agree that in order to build a strong, healthy body you need to exercise. The word *exercise* implies movement: strengthening, toning, stretching, and working your body. Sadhana Yoga teaches to strive for a balance in all aspects of life, including exercise.

You can build your body through aerobic exercise, muscle resistance exercise, stretching exercise, and proper diet. If you choose not to engage in any of these categories, then you will never succeed at building your body to its full potential. If you partake in only a few of these four categories, you will have some success, yet you will still lack in achieving your full potential. Through the Sadhana Yoga system you will embrace all four categories and achieve a well-balanced, healthy, strong, and flexible body.

AEROBIC EXERCISE

Aerobic exercise includes any exercise that puts stress on working your heart and lungs. This would include any exercise which gets you breathing hard and increases your heart rate to its maximum sustained beat. Ideally, you need to maintain this state for a sustained period of time, depending on your general health. Experts recommend getting at least a minimum of fifteen minutes of aerobic activity daily.

There are many ways to fulfill your aerobic needs, such as biking, fast walking, running, hiking, swimming, dancing, and many other movement activities. These are all excellent ways to improve your aerobic conditioning; however, these other activities can often leave you tired and stiff with sore muscles. In yoga exercise you consume more oxygen than you expend energy. In other aerobic activities you expend more energy than you consume oxygen. For this reason, after a properly executed yoga practice, you have a euphoric energized feeling which lasts for many hours, with less chance of creating sore muscles.

You may have experienced or have heard about spontaneously experiencing "euphoria" or "the zone" in peak performance or in sports. The physical practice of Sadhana Yoga is one way of easily awakening to this effortless and energized state. Yoga exercise can be aerobic if you choose a routine which challenges your heart and respiratory system. I endorse supplementing your yoga practice with other moderate aerobic exercise. The addition of another aerobic activity will only help you in embracing a more full spectrum of Sadhana Yoga.

MUSCLE-RESISTANCE EXERCISE

Muscle-resistance exercise strengthens muscles with less emphasis on heart rate and respiratory functions. Try to incorporate at least 20 minutes of quality muscle-resistance exercise every other day. Quality muscle-resistance exercise refers to challenging your muscles. Because muscle-resistance exercise usually targets one specific muscle group, you need to focus on different areas of your body with each separate workout. This cross-training within muscle resistance usually covers the main muscle groups of legs, arms, and abdominal muscles. One day you might choose to work your legs with hiking, leg presses, or weights, the next workout would focus on your arms with push-ups or weight training, and the following workout the focus would be on abdominal muscles with sit-ups.

Sometimes aerobic and muscle-resistance exercise can go hand and hand, in that it is possible to have one exercise accomplish both categories. Yoga is this sort of exercise: it can provide a major source of muscle-resistance exercise for all areas of your body while increasing your heart rate. Yoga becomes a muscle-resistance exercise because you are lifting your own body weight, doing abdominal work, as well as isometrics. The results can be a full and complete strengthening of your whole body. So unlike aerobic exercise, where you may want to supplement your yoga with additional aerobic exercise to meet the daily criteria, this is not necessary with muscle-resistance exercise. In this system, yoga will have your muscle-resistance training covered.

STRETCHING EXERCISE

Isolated stretching exercise implies the lengthening of the muscles, joints, and tendons without emphasis on your respiratory system, circulatory system, or strengthening of muscles. Pure stretching is different from yoga exercise, yet yoga exercise definitely involves stretching. Yoga differs from simple stretching as it also embraces techniques of synchronized breathing, counter stretching, the mind-body connection, and proper sequencing of yoga postures. Stretching your muscles with yoga helps to release tension from your muscles and creates more supple joints and tendons. Ideally, you should strive to stretch for a minimum of thirty to forty-five minutes two or three times a week. This also depends on what else you are doing in your life; if you are very physically active, you might want to stretch more. However, this stretching requirement is easily met during each yoga practice.

FUELING YOUR BODY

Sadhana Yoga also stresses the importance of a proper diet. You will learn that the food you choose can greatly enhance the effects of the vital life force. The human body is a wonderful machine, provided you supply it with the proper fuel in the form of nutritious food.

Merging Your Mind

The goal of Sadhana Yoga is to create a mind-body connection. Through mastering the postures and links, you will become aware of your every movement as you draw lines of energy from the Earth right through your body. Let you body and mind flow freely as one unit, and your yoga will follow with flowing grace. As you feel this sacred movement from your heart, you will desire only to be in the moment, creating your own paradise within. Visualize the energy moving through your yoga practice, as if you have no body, only an energy field seeking the natural flow of the universe. Much like a dancer, or musician, let your yoga practice tell a beautiful story, as it reflects your inner harmony.

This mind-body connection is the ultimate in yoga practice: a true experience of *prana*. You can greatly enhance your mind-body connection by incorporating specific breathing techniques and the lessons of sense withdrawal and mind focus to help you surrender to the natural flow.

THE SOOTHING TOUCH OF BREATH

The single most important aspect of your life is breath. The science and art of yoga breathing is one of the most valuable tools to reconnect you with the vital life force. One of the primary requirements to participating in Sadhana Yoga is to learn proper breathing. These techniques will supply you with greater energy and strength, deeper relaxation, more mental clarity, and peace of mind. Proper breathing also aids your circulatory system in supplying fresh oxygenated blood to every area of your body. Yoga breathing will also cleanse toxins from your lungs and enhance their performance.

THE POWER SENSE WITHDRAWAL

Sense withdrawal is a very necessary step for an enhanced yoga practice. You cannot build a house without a good foundation, and sense withdrawal is a great internal foundation to build wonderful external effects in your yoga and throughout your life. With sense withdrawal you turn your attention inward and focus on your breathing techniques, body alignment, and internal muscular locks. If your body and mind are totally connected within every movement in your yoga practice, then you can use this same technique to assist you through your whole life.

SOOTHING YOUR SPIRIT

Proper relaxation plays an important part in Sadhana Yoga. Relaxation can be divided into three separate categories: rest, sleep, and leisure time with nature. Your body needs rest in order to totally recover from physical and mental work. Along the same lines, the yogic techniques to ensure getting quality sleep is just as important as yoga exercise. Many people never really get a complete restful night's sleep: through your yoga practice you will learn how to embrace quality sleep. Meditation is another wonderful tool to help sooth, relax, and focus your mind.

The main aspect which separates Sadhana Yoga from other exercise programs, and other styles of yoga, is that this system soothes your spirit. After just a few weeks of this new practice you will have a new positive outlook on life, feeling content and at peace. In today's fast-paced society, we all need a little tender loving care and this program will embrace you with open arms and console your inner spirit.

Surrender to the Flow

After you have embraced proper breathing, sense withdrawal, and achieved a relaxed state, you can begin practicing yoga postures without focusing on the physical actions and simply go with the flow. This concept, called *dhyana*, (meaning "meditation in motion") is the point in yoga practice when you have achieved the mind-body connection. You have reached an effortless mastery of posture and movement while embracing all the aspects of quality yoga practice, as they are in sync with the natural energy flow of all life. Ultimately, you will become one with the wind, the trees, the mountains, and the whole universe, completely absorbed into your yoga energy flow.

For some people, achieving this level of *dhyana* will come easily with practice. For others it may take a little more perseverance. The secret is in letting go, yet at the same time remaining focused and mastering your practice, surrendering to the energy flow. Instead of thinking of dragging yourself through your yoga practice, go with the natural flow of energy and let your yoga softly lead you.

The Spiritual Element of Yoga Practice

Spirituality can and does mean different things to different people. Religion does not have to play a part in spirituality, yet for some religion is spirituality. Through the Sadhana Yoga system, there is no designated religious connection, and this program will only serve to enhance your own beliefs.

To some, spirituality means closeness to nature and creating a feeling of inner peace. To others, spirituality embraces a faith and respect in some greater power that encompasses all that is good. Still, others believe that spirituality is something that is felt deep within and cannot be explained with mere words.

In the philosophy of Sadhana Yoga, true spirituality is to embrace kindness, compassion, and selfless giving. At the same time to hold peace in your heart and become a vehicle for all that is good to channel through your body and mind. When you master Sadhana Yoga, you reflect spirituality through telling a story with your yoga practice and flow with the energy of life.

STAYING CONNECTED

It may seem hard enough to practice yoga, let alone to embrace a spiritual element. Yet there is a seemingly timeless saying which indicates others have experienced the same difficulties as you: "Seek out the infinite answers to the universe, and they will surely elude you." Calm your mind, find inner peace, and the answers to the infinite universe will seek you out.

When beginning your yoga routine, the spiritual elements will gradually enter into your practice. Don't try too hard, just gently remind yourself to embrace a spiritual element in your practice. Let your yoga become a very sacred journey, filled with wonderful experiences. Let yoga become a sanctuary, a place where all is good. Let your best qualities surface from your spirit and become one with the flow of your yoga and all life. Still your body, quiet your mind, and listen to the heartbeat of Earth, as you flow with the universe in a timeless moment.

Pulling It All Together

Once you have begun your journey with Sadhana Yoga, you have planted the seeds of success. You can then tap into this valuable resource throughout your daily life. Many students of yoga turn off this great energy once they leave the yoga studio. Don't make this mistake! With Sadhana Yoga I encourage you to draw from this vast well of rich positive energy every day. Don't just become a student of yoga; let your yoga become a student of yours, as you channel this energy into everything you do. You now have the infinite power and soothing touch of nature's energy at your disposal. Along with this you have inner harmony, strength, intelligence, and grace. Train your yoga to help you whenever possible, let the natural energy of the universe flow free throughout your body and mind.

Some days, as you drag yourself through your routine, you will find your yoga is only exercise. Then there will be other times when you feel so magically connected and focused, it will make you want to cry with joy and tell everyone you see. On the days you are in sync with the natural flow of energy, you will definitely know it! The most important thing is to be kind, have patience, cut yourself some slack, and believe in your own true self. In time you will have more magical connected practices and less nonconnected practices.

Adapting Sadhana Yoga Flow to Your Practice

Become a humble beginner and empty your cup
Open your heart, collect your soul, and create a universe

Not long ago, an aspiring *yogi* or *yogini* such as yourself would have had to travel great distances over frozen mountains and across blazing deserts to find a worthy teacher. Upon finding this teacher, you would then be subject to sleeping in the snow, fasting for thirty days, practicing your yoga in a room full of poisonous snakes, or enduring many other physical and mental tests. These trials were simply to determine if you were worthy of being a serious student. Your choices of yoga styles were also greatly limited:

you could choose between one *guru* teaching postures and another *guru* teaching meditation.

Now that yoga practice seems to have reached just about every inch of the world, the availability and variety of styles has grown as well. The good news is you no longer have to climb a mountain to find a great teacher, and there are a wide variety of yoga styles to choose from.

I have great respect and appreciation for all styles of yoga practice and for those who have endeavored to teach the various styles. Because of the efforts of the many individuals who practice and teach yoga, this science and healing art has touched our society in a very positive and nurturing way.

In the first known yoga text, the Indian sage Patanjali categorized yoga as an eight-limb path. The trunk that connected this eight-limbed path represents the common ground that all yoga teachings embrace. All styles of yoga are aimed at improving the quality of life through a series of physical and mental challenges. Patanjali further classified yoga into sixteen separate categories, or systems. Each of the sixteen separate categories were represented as petals on a lotus flower, as the flower floated effortlessly on the quiet pond of life.

THE EIGHT LIMBS OF YOGA

1. *Yama*—Abstinences:
   a. *Ahimsa*—Embrace peace and non-violence
   b. *Satya*—Be truthful and honest in all ways
   c. *Asteya*—Refrain from stealing and cheating
   d. *Brahmacharya*—Maintain integrity of intimate relationships
   e. *Aparigraha*—Refrain from hoarding: be free from the bonds of materialism

2. *Niyama*—Observances:
   a. *Saucha*—Strive for purity in body, mind, and spirit
   b. *Santosa*—Embrace contentment within simplicity, and feel tranquility
   c. *Tapas*—Endure work and hardship in exchange for an improved body and mind
   d. *Svadhyaya*—Embrace self-study and always see yourself as a student
   e. *Isvara*—Be humble in the presence of the supreme being, or energy

3. *Asana*—Postures
   The practice of the sacred yoga postures for physical and mental health

4. *Pranayama*—Breathing
   The science, art, and practice of enhanced breathing techniques

5. *Pratyahara*—Sense Withdrawal
   Withdrawal of your senses in order to gaze inward and maintain clear focus

6. *Dharana*—Concentration
   Learn to concentrate by focusing all your energy on a particular area of thought

7. *Dhyana*—Meditation
   Gain complete control over your mind with sustained, effortless, and relaxed intellect

8. *Samadhi*—Self-Realization
   To reach enlightenment, shed the ego and become one with the universe

Philosophy and Background of Yoga

The basic philosophy of yoga is centered around creating a balance between your physical, mental, and spiritual health. This balance can be achieved through disciplines of physical and mental exercise, breathing techniques, deep relaxation, and following a pure diet. The end result is a connection with the natural flow of energy in the universe.

Wise sages and *gurus* thought that the answers to the questions on how humans could live a healthier and more productive life were found in the hands of Mother Nature. From studying different animals, these wise sages came to the conclusion that there was a balance of strength and softness within all creatures and within nature itself. In time their teachings evolved into a practical system that was handed down from teacher to student over thousands of years. The connection of an improved diet, along with techniques of fasting and the evolution of yoga postures and mental training techniques, formed the system that we now refer to as *Yoga*. This system created a positive direction for all humans to greatly enhance their physical, mental, and spiritual health.

The Similarities Found in All Yoga

The most noted skill of all *Hatha* Yoga styles is the mastery of the yoga postures. The individual postures are called *asanas*, which translates as meaning "position comfortably held." When done correctly, each *asana* creates a very powerful source of vital life-force energy.

Most styles also train their students on the important elements of deep concentration, mind focus, positive thought, and gaining control over your restless mind through relaxation and meditation techniques. Most styles of yoga teach a sense of connection within body, mind, and spirit. Most styles of yoga also focus on reaching an ultimate goal of self-enlightenment, self-realization, or true inner peace with one's self and the whole universe.

The branch of yoga most widely practiced today is really a combination between the traditional branches of *Hatha* Yoga and *Raja* Yoga. *Hatha* Yoga is basically increasing your health and *Raja* Yoga is mastery of the mind. The combination of the two categories translates as meaning, a balanced physical and mental health, a union between *yin* and *yang*, or masculine and feminine. The goal of *Hatha* Yoga combined with *Raja* Yoga is to achieve a body of perfect health and strength, a mind which is relaxed, yet sharp and intelligent, and to embrace peace and harmony in your heart leading to an unbridled vision of all life.

The Different Styles of Yoga Practice

Within this broader category of *Hatha*/*Raja* Yoga, there are dozens of different practices. While all *Hatha* Yoga styles are based on the order and repetition of the *asanas*, what makes each philosophy unique is the choice between the various postures, how long they are held for, how to enter and exit each posture, and what type of breathing they are accompanied by.

The Hard and Soft Sides of Hatha Yoga

Further, you can loosely divide all styles of *Hatha* yoga practice between hard and soft styles. Hard styles traditionally take more work, are more physically demanding, build your muscles more, and can be semi-aerobic. Hard styles also instill a greater feeling of self-confidence and inner strength. Soft styles take less energy and are focused more on stretching and relaxing rather than endurance, aerobics, and increased strength. Soft styles embrace a greater feeling of inner peace and mental clarity. As in everything else, there are exceptions to this rule: hard yoga can be soft and soft yoga can definitely be hard. If you only practice a soft-style yoga, you are missing something on the holistic spectrum of energy. The same holds true if you only practice hard forms, again you are missing something on the holistic spectrum of energy.

The following are some of the main styles of yoga being taught today. You can probably find a class in one or more of these varieties in major cities and towns across the country.

ANASURA YOGA—Founded by John Friend in 1997. John had a deep background training in the Iyengar tradition and has used these concepts along with many great ideas of his own to found a new system of *Anasura* Yoga. The Sanskrit word *anasura* translates as meaning "flowing with grace." This system is grounded in the philosophy of embracing all the concepts of correct alignment, yet encouraging students to connect to the spiritual purpose behind the posture as well. This system has three governing properties: (1) attitude, (2) alignment, and (3) action. In a very short time *Anasura* Yoga has become quite popular.

ASHTANGA YOGA—Co-founded by K. Pattabhi Jois and his teacher Krishnamacharya in the 1930s, and introduced in America in the mid 1970s by two American *yogis*, David Williams and Norman Allen. Pattabhi Jois believed this system was a part of the original *Yoga Sutras* of Patanjali and therefore named it *Ashtanga* Yoga, meaning "the eight-limbed path." This is definitely a physically hard form of yoga practice. It has a vigorous linking system, with an emphasis on strength, endurance, and repetitions during practice. This system can be very aerobic and challenging to the muscles for even a professional athlete. At present there are six levels of *Ashtanga* Yoga practice, although the beginners level is usually enough for most people. With the help of great instructors like my brother, David Swenson, this system is very popular throughout the world today

BIKRAM YOGA—Founded by Bikram Choudhury. Bikram had some health problems and through the avenue of yoga found specific postures, practiced in a very hot room, assisted in his recovery. Bikram introduced his hot yoga to the stars in Hollywood in the 1970s and now has a large following all over the country. In Bikram Yoga the yoga room or studio will be heated to 105 degrees. The philosophy is with more heat you are more flexible, have less chance of injury, and sweat off more toxins. Within this style you will practice only twenty-six postures, hold each posture twice, once for 30 seconds and the second time for 60 seconds.

IYENGAR YOGA—Founded by B.K.S. Iyengar, who first brought his style of yoga to America in 1966. Iyengar Yoga can be hard or soft style, depending on your level of practice and the individual teacher. This style is known for its great emphasis on structural alignment and use of props during yoga practice. In an Iyengar class you would generally practice fewer different yoga postures in a session, but hold each of the postures longer and receive a very detailed evaluation of your posture execution. Iyengar has been the inspiration for thousands of students in opening hundreds of yoga centers in many countries worldwide.

KRIPALU YOGA—Founded by Swami Kripalu, who was the spiritual teacher of Yogi Amrit Desai. Amrit Desai founded the Kripalu Yoga Center in Lennox, Massachusetts in the late 1970s. This is basically soft-form yoga with a holistic outlook. This style also embraces healing through diet and internal cleansing techniques. The Sanskrit word *kripal* translates as meaning "compassion" or "mercy," and this compassion is the general theme of Kripalu Yoga. In this philosophy your spirit will grow when it is watered with compassion. This center has become one of the largest centers for yoga and holistic health in the U.S.

KUNDALINI YOGA—Founded by Yogi Bhajan who first introduced this style in America in the late 1960s. It is now taught all over the world. The philosophy of *Kundalini* Yoga covers an awakening of the mystical dormant *kundalini* energy, which resides at the base of your spine. The Sanskrit word *kundalini* is derived from the root *kundal* which indicates a coiled lock of hair from a loved one. In *Kundalini* Yoga, the practice of awakening the *kundalini* energy is symbolic of uncoiling the lock of hair. This is basically a soft-form practice with a great emphasis on awakening the dormant universal energies within your body through the recitation of *mantras*, warm-up exercises, specific yoga postures, deep relaxation, and meditation.

POWER YOGA—First founded by Beryl Bender Birch and Tom Birch in the early 1990s. Beryl and Tom taught great yoga in the New York City area for many years before discovering the powerful system of *Ashtanga* Yoga. Power Yoga is actually *Ashtanga* Yoga with a different marketing slant in order to reach a larger group of students. Beryl's book greatly influenced the recent popularity of *Ashtanga* Yoga. Today Power Yoga does not aptly describe a particular style of yoga since the name Power Yoga can mean different things to different instructors. For example, Brian Kest and Baron Baptiste, two noted Power Yoga instructors, each has a somewhat different approach. However, their common ground is that you will always get a hard physical workout during Power Yoga.

SIVANANDA YOGA AND INTEGRAL YOGA—*Sivananda* Yoga, founded by Swami Vishnu Devananda, and Integral Yoga, founded by Swami Satchidananda, are two separate styles of yoga practice, yet are both basically soft-form styles. In these styles you will practice a set structure with a variety of yoga postures, meditation, and some guidelines for healthy living. These two separate styles of yoga are very soothing, gentle, and warming to the spirit. *Sivananda* and Integral styles were some of the first types of yoga introduced in America. These styles are very mellow, relaxing, and low energy. *Sivananda* Yoga is one of the world's largest yoga schools in existence today.

VINI YOGA—Founded by T.K.V. Desikachar, inspired by his father Sri T. Krishnamacharya. T. Krishnamacharya was also the teacher and *guru* of B.K.S. Iyengar, T.K.V. Desikachar, and K. Pattabhi Jois. In Sanskrit the word *vini* translates as meaning "individual, gradual, or special." *Vini* Yoga recognizes the unique qualities of each individual. This is basically a soft-form style of yoga practice. One of the most well-renowned yoga masters of the last century, T. Krishnamacharya taught on a very individual basis, adjusting a yoga posture so that it fit each participant. Of all the styles, this one clearly incorporates both *Hatha* and *Raja* Yoga into its practice.

VINYASA YOGA—This is a generic term used to loosely describe a hybrid version of *Ashtanga* Yoga, or simply the use of any *vinyasa* between postures in several different yoga styles. There is no overall holistic structure to posture sequence, and it will usually be taught differently by each individual teacher.

THE SADHANA YOGA FLOW PROGRAM

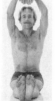

Sadhana Yoga is comparable to all other existing yoga practices. It uses many of the same postures and familiar techniques of breathing. Yet with most of the yoga styles mentioned, each of the postures is completed by holding the pose for a specific amount of time, followed by a moment of rest. This creates a segmented energy pattern and, ultimately, a loss of energy: each time you end a yoga posture you are breaking the current of energy, and much of the *prana* created is lost.

In order to derive the maximum energy from your yoga practice, you need to connect the yoga postures together. The Sadhana Yoga system is based on new innovative connective links that continue the flow of energy from one *asana* to the next. These energy-compatible flowing links are called *vinyasas,* and serve as the "electrical wiring" that connects the energy from posture to posture.

There are other yoga practices that include some generic linking connections between postures; most of these systems were directly or indirectly derived from *Ashtanga Yoga*. From this introduction of linking postures together other similar styles have emerged, including the now-popular Power Yoga. Other hard-form styles use a few generic transitional movements throughout the practice that connect various yoga postures, this method does not take into account the energy flow of each individual yoga posture. Sadhana Yoga teaches separate connecting movements for each individual yoga posture, along with a few base *vinyasas*, to teach energy lines, taking into consideration the energy flow of each separate posture.

Also, the physically demanding connecting movements found in other hard-form styles are considered by many to be very difficult, rigid, and rough. They can cause a scattered energy flow and worse, injury to the joints. In Sadhana Yoga the connecting movements are strength building, very smooth, circular in motion, graceful, and flow like a soft poetic dance. These connecting movements are easy on the body and can be performed no matter what your level of fitness or previous yoga experience. Sadhana Yoga uses a variety of different *vinyasas*, each based on the energy flow of the individual yoga postures.

The most exciting aspect of developing Sadhana Yoga is that it was created to be a universal *vinyasa* system, which means that you can use these concepts with any other style of practice. No matter what type of yoga you already do, Sadhana Yoga can enhance its performance. What's more, it caters to all levels of yoga practice, from beginners through advanced students. It can be very challenging to even the most advanced yoga student.

The Sadhana Yoga system is designed to affect every area of your body, with nothing left untouched. It combines the best of both the hard-form and soft-form worlds as it reflects softness as strength. It endorses the use of proper yoga sequencing for enhanced comfort and energy flow. Sadhana Yoga also embraces proper diet and body-cleansing techniques with additional teachings on how yoga can help to influence your whole life in a positive way.

Outwardly the *vinyasa* creates a beautiful flow of continuous energy. Your yoga practice between postures will resemble a continuous soft-flowing dance that will in time become graceful and effortless. After just a few weeks of practicing Sadhana Yoga, you will notice improvements in all your physical activities: everything will become more fluid for you in all areas of sports, games, recreation, and hobbies.

Your mind is a reflection of your physical actions therefore changes in your body also affect your emotional state. Once you have embraced Sadhana Yoga, you will experience a more focused mind and feel a direct connection with the natural flow of the vital life force. As you notice more physical energy, you will also notice an increase in mental energy as well, whether you are reading books, organizing your thoughts, working, or just relaxing with a friend or loved one. You will develop a sense of well-being, greater self-confidence, and find yourself in tune with positive thoughts. Everyone will love to be around you as you find it easier to communicate and touch the hearts of others.

ENHANCE YOUR YOGA PRACTICE WITH FLOW

Whether you are a first-time yoga student, a seasoned regular, or a yoga teacher, you will find that Sadhana Yoga can greatly enhance your yoga practice and your whole life. If you 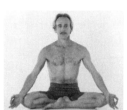 are already practicing some form of yoga, you can easily adapt concepts of Sadhana Yoga into your existing practice. The first concept you will learn is the breathing and concentration techniques for each separate flowing link; this will have a great effect on the outcome of your movement. Then pick a yoga routine that is not over your head; start out with something you feel comfortable with. Once you understand the instructions, you will start connecting your postures together with my unique *vinyasa* flow. Finally, you will incorporate the mind-body connection with your energy flow. You will be aware of the energy lines you are drawing within the movement of your own flowing links.

The flowing links will not change the way you practice your individual yoga postures, or the length of time you hold each posture. Remember, any kind of yoga practice is very beneficial, and even if you do not use a flowing connection you will derive benefits from practicing yoga. However, if you incorporate the Sadhana flowing links into your yoga practice, you will discover greater relaxation, focus, strength, and inner peace from your very first time. I suggest you do an experiment! Go through your yoga postures without using any of my flowing links to connect your postures. After your yoga practice, write down how you feel physically and mentally. Then read through the instructions in the following sections, and the next time you practice your yoga, do the same routine using my suggested flowing connections. Once again, write down how you feel afterward: the results will be amazing.

Regardless of your previous experience with yoga, I suggest starting this practice with the beginner routines. As you improve, you will quickly progress at your own pace to the more challenging routines, all the while harnessing the strong fluid movements and continuous lines of *prana* energy.

If you are completely new to yoga, I suggest that you begin by practicing the various yoga postures without the flowing links until you gain some confidence and feel comfortable in the different poses. This does not mean you should not practice the flow because you are a beginner; by all means indulge yourself if you feel that you are ready. However, if you first gain a little self-confidence, then your flow will feel more comfortable, yet powerful and energizing as your yoga takes on the essence of the blissful softness and incredible strength of nature.

AS A BEGINNER TO YOGA—After a few weeks of concentrating on the yoga postures, you will start to feel the energy flow within each individual pose. Your body will also have time to adapt to this new exercise movement, and you will feel more comfortable with yoga in general. Work on your deep, complete yoga breathing and become familiar with the order of posture sequencing. Then you can start adding the flowing links between your yoga postures.

PRACTICING ENERGY FLOW IN ALL THINGS

Over the years I realized there is a natural energy flow to all things in the universe, not just yoga postures. This flow encompasses everything from diet and nutrition to the way you think and communicate. Sadhana Yoga reconnects with this natural flow of energy as you achieve your ultimate physical, mental, and spiritual health.

Moving Meditation for the Ultimate Flow

Your practice of yoga is for you and ultimately it should be something you feel very comfortable with. As in all things, you've got to start somewhere! Do you remember the first time you rode a bicycle, drove a car, or went surfing? It seemed like an enormous task to master any of these activities: I'm sure you felt that you would never find them relaxing or comfortable. Luckily, once you understood the basics, all these activities just became second nature.

You will find the same to be true of your Sadhana Yoga practice: in time all the details will become second nature and you can just move with the natural flow of energy, like a surfer riding the energy of a beautiful wave. I remember when I was a very rank beginner in my yoga practice: I tried too hard, fixating on all the minor details. I really had a miserable time at my yoga, and it was more like work than something relaxing and enjoyable. Then one day I just thought, to heck with all the details, I am just going to do some yoga outdoors for fun. It was a wonderful experience, being able to free my spirit and practice yoga. Gradually I embraced all the concepts and details of good yoga practice. Today my yoga practice feels very free-flowing, comfortable, and with a balance of strength and softness. Physically I am amazingly strong, mentally I am very focused, and spiritually I am at peace with myself and with my place in the universe.

The ultimate in Sadhana Yoga *asana* practice is to embrace all your connecting movements as a moving meditation. As you gain confidence, strength, and greater awareness with your practice, you will strive toward having razor-sharp focus in all aspects of your movements, yet with effortless fluidity. Your practice will float like a cloud, directed by the energy of the wind (referring to your breath and *prana*). At this point you will let your mind flow free, visualizing where you are going with your movements as your body follows your mind's lead with effortless silence on the eternal journey along the stream of life.

PART II

————

THE SADHANA

YOGA PRACTICE

_____

THREE

PREPARING FOR SADHANA
YOGA FLOW

Thought creates energy
As prana *dances with youth*
In the ageless mind

Yoga is a very individualized practice. Unlike competitive activities where you strive to become the single winner, in yoga, everyone is a winner. The goal in yoga is to find a routine which works best for you. Over time this routine may change to something completely different as you evolve with your practice. This growth, plus adding the other elements of Sadhana Yoga (meditation and diet), will lead to the ultimate yoga experience.

I often refer to physically demanding yoga practice as hard flow and the less physically demanding as soft flow. Through the practice of Sadhana Yoga you will find both softness and strength within each individual routine. If you want to work hard and really build your muscles, try a hard-flow workout. If you want to increase flexibility and have a lighter form of exercise, try a soft-flow workout. You can even structure a little of both into one routine. However, speeding up your routine in order to turn up the heat does not create a harder workout. It will only sap your energy and distract you from achieving a yogic state of mind.

In order to begin your practice, there are certain choices you need to make, as well as key techniques that need to be studied. The first decision is choosing how strenuous and challenging a workout you would like to have. Control over the amount of physical work within your yoga routine is achieved through four variables: the choices of yoga postures, how you practice your postures, length of time holding the postures, and your choice of *vinyasa*.

Choice of Yoga Postures

The yoga postures themselves have a great deal to do with the level of challenge in your practice. Some postures are very easy to embrace without having to defy gravity or balance on your arms. On the other hand, if you want a greater physical challenge, you need to do something other than laying flat on your back in the Corpse Posture in order to get your internal turbo boost charged.

How You Practice Your Yoga Postures

The manor in which you practice your yoga postures also has an impact on the level of physical challenge in your routine. For example, if you are practicing a very challenging standing posture like Warrior II, you can make it even more challenging by sinking deeper into your lunge. Or you can make the posture less challenging by backing off a bit and conserving your energy for another posture.

Length of Time

The length of time you choose to stay in an individual yoga posture can also affect the challenge level. Even a nonstrenuous posture such as Tree Posture can be very demanding if you hold this posture for more than ten minutes. On the other hand, if you are practicing a difficult arm balance like the Crane Posture and only hold the posture for a few seconds, then you have not created much of a challenge.

Choice of Vinyasa

Your choice of *vinyasa* (the connection between postures) can quite dramatically affect your level of physical challenge. I will give you several choices between more or less challenging *vinyasas* to connect your postures together. The more challenging *vinyasa* will work your muscles to a much greater degree as you are resisting your own body weight against gravity, and in some cases the more challenging *vinyasa* is a more involved movement. For example, you may move from lying on the floor all the way to standing and back to the floor again, all as one *vinyasa*. In the less challenging *vinyasa*, the muscle resistance factor is much lower, and in some cases the movements are less involved and very subtle, like lifting your arms up over you head and back down again.

Evaluating Your Needs

In order to get the most out of any yoga practice, you first have to evaluate your motivations. Here are a set of questions that will help determine what type of yoga practice is right for you.

  • *What kind of physical condition are you in and do you have any injuries or
    limitations?*

Your physical condition is always a factor in getting started in yoga or any other physical program. Sadhana Yoga is noncompetitive, and no matter what your age, shape, or size, you will benefit. Whether you are completely out of shape or a contending Olympic athlete, you can find sanctuary with this practice.

If you have not exercised for more than six months, it is a good idea to check with your physician before embarking on your yoga journey. Then take it slow, pick beginner routines, and do light cross-training with other forms of exercise. If you have any injuries you should be attentive of this in your own practice and let your teacher know which area of your body has problems. Many times simple adjustments to the postures or props will assist you in overcoming your injuries. Other times you might need to avoid certain yoga postures altogether.

- *Are you looking for something nonstrenuous with a very light pace that focuses mostly on relaxation and stretching, or do you want a really good physical workout as well?*

There are many different reasons to practice yoga, and each student comes to the studio with different needs. Your motives will also change over time as your practice evolves. If your daily work is very strenuous, you might want to take it easy with your yoga and focus on creating a warm, gentle practice to rejuvenate your physical and mental reserves. When my job involved lots of physical activity, the last thing I wanted to do at the end of the day was a strenuous workout.

Now I often find myself for days in a row sitting on airplanes, driving in traffic, typing on my computer, and giving lectures. After several days or weeks of this lifestyle I often seek the more powerful avenue of yoga practice to really work my muscles, break into a good sweat, and at the same time release stress and tension.

You do not have to choose one practice style over the other: you might want to incorporate both aspects into one practice, or do as I sometimes do, practice Soft Flow one day and Hard Flow the next. Through the program of Sadhana Yoga you are in control and can choose which is in your own best interest.

- *Are you a newcomer, beginner, intermediate, or advanced student of yoga?*

Your background and experience with yoga also has a very profound impact on what type of practice you choose to embrace. As a beginner you might want to just test the water before you jump in for a swim. Learn the basics of Sadhana Yoga and see how you feel. In this case you would benefit by first studying the foundation for yoga and then trying out a Soft-Flow beginner routine.

For intermediate students, it is still a good idea to review the foundations of Sadhana Yoga. You may learn something new and then seek a moderate routine, work on your technique, alignment, and fluid motion of *vinyasa*. There is no shame in backing down and practicing a simpler routine; take a practice vacation to enjoy familiar ground.

If you're an advanced student, this is a wonderful opportunity to refine your every move while still discovering a new style of yoga. Again, it is best to review the foundations of Sadhana Yoga; after all, this is a brand-new style, and many small changes can make a profound impact on your overall practice. You might want to seek a very challenging aspect of practice, and with this I do not only refer to the physical avenue. A challenge can be practicing a beautiful flow of *vinyasa*, holding postures a bit longer, refining your breath, and creating a very intimate mind-body connection. Ultimately you want your practice to become a moving meditation and connect with the natural flow of energy, not only within yourself, but throughout your whole life.

- *How much time do you have to practice daily and how many times a week?*

We all have very different lifestyles and need to make adjustments in order to find time to treat ourselves to the gift of yoga. Perhaps you can only practice for 45 minutes, two times a week, or maybe you are lucky enough to be able to practice 2½ hours every day. Whatever amount of time you can devote to yoga practice, make sure that it is quality time by treating yourself with the ultimate respect and savoring the moment.

If you have lots of time for yoga, make sure to take a break now and then. Sometimes too much yoga can drain your energy, cause injury, and result in a progress block where you can't break new ground. It is also a good idea to rotate between hard- and soft-form practice, and indoor and outdoor practice. Seek mastery over your simplistic moves and focus on the spiritual element of your practice rather than just turning yoga into another physical workout.

- *Are you practicing by yourself or in a class setting?*

Practicing in a studio has the advantage of group support and energy. Practicing alone gives you privacy and better internal focus. When I first started practicing yoga in the 1960s, anyone practicing yoga was practicing alone. I never had the luxury of studios and group practice, so I found my energy more centered on peace, tranquility, and contemplation. You have many more options these days, and I suggest that you seek both ends of the spectrum, with solitude on certain days and group support and energy on others.

IF YOU ARE LOOKING FOR A HARD-FLOW WORKOUT

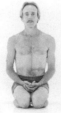

When yoga was first introduced to the Western world, the idea of achieving a good physical workout from yoga practice was literally unheard of. However, since the early seventies with the introduction of *Ashtanga* Yoga, several other styles have emerged which are based on a very physical workout, which I consider Hard-Flow yoga. If you are looking to challenge your aerobic capabilities as well as build muscles, Sadhana Yoga can create this type of Hard-Flow workout.

Getting an Aerobic Workout with Sadhana Yoga

Sadhana Yoga can be considered a semi-aerobic workout if you choose the more challenging *vinyasa* approach to practice with a more challenging routine, which works your heart and respiratory system. Aerobic qualities vary from one individual to the next. Getting your heart rate up to at least 70 percent of its maximum power and sustaining this for at least 15 minutes is the true measure of what is considered to be an aerobic activity. If you are a marathon runner you will have to work harder to get your aerobic workout level than someone who is out of shape.

The good thing is you can easily meet the minimum requirements for an aerobic workout within Sadhana Yoga, but to do this you have to challenge yourself. Lying down in the Corpse Posture or resting in a Forward Bend will not get you where you want to go. However, remember that you don't have to race through your routine in order to get more of an aerobic workout in yoga. Getting an aerobic yoga workout will be interlaced with the same postures used for an anaerobic workout.

Discovering Muscle Resistance Exercise with Sadhana Yoga

If you are seeking muscle-resistance exercise, you can find more than enough within Sadhana Yoga to satisfy even an Olympic athlete. There are several factors which influence the strength-building aspects of your yoga practice. Muscle-resistance exercise is achieved in yoga by supporting your own body weight within yoga postures, moving your own body weight from one posture to another, partner adjustment work, and through isometric exercise within your practice in the form of the yoga postures and the connecting links.

Each yoga posture, or *asana*, ranges within the spectrum of muscle-resistance quality. For example, a Seated Forward Bend takes very little strength to complete, while a Handstand is very physically demanding. In the Seated Forward Bend you are getting very little muscle-resistance exercise, mostly just stretching the back side of your body. On the other hand, in the Handstand you are pushing your own body weight up over your head, much like weight lifting. You can choose the number of strenuous postures to work into your routine, thereby controlling the amount of muscle-resistance exercise within your yoga practice.

Isometric exercise is the method of resisting one muscle against another. In many yoga postures you will use what I call opposition of stretch. For example, if you are stretching forward in the Expanded Foot Posture, at the same time you are moving your arms backward in opposition of stretch: this opposite movement creates muscle resistance.

One of the key factors in determining just how much of a muscle-resistance work-out you will get is the *vinyasa*, or the linking movements between your yoga postures. You can choose a *vinyasa* which is very physically demanding (Hot *vinyasa*), or you can choose a *vinyasa* which is very low energy (Cool *vinyasa*). The difference between these choices is dramatic, and again, the choice is up to you. You can choose the hotter *vinyasas*, the cooler *vinyasas*, or use a bit of both.

How fast you move through your *vinyasa* also affects the muscle resistance and iso-metric qualities of your practice. Surprisingly, the slower you move in your practice, the greater the quality of muscle-resistance workout. When you move at a slower rate in your *vinyasa*, you remain in the muscle-resistance area longer than when you're moving very quickly. For example, if two students practiced a Sun Salutation, the student who moved slower and finished last would achieve a greater muscle-resistance workout. The one who moved quicker would be running on momentum and sacrificing slow deep breathing, a tranquil atmosphere, and the loss of energy.

As in any muscle-resistance activity, gradually work up to more challenging, strength-building yoga routines. As a newcomer to yoga the best thing to do is take it easy, try out a beginner-level routine and see how you feel. Then gradually increase your challenge and you will find that you enjoy your yoga practice much more.

IF YOU ARE LOOKING FOR A SOFT-FLOW WORKOUT

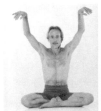

Envision a peaceful river winding through the countryside. As gentle as this river seems, you know that it is strong enough to create its own path. What you are observing is the marriage between softness and strength. Sadhana Yoga embraces this concept and manifests it within the Soft-Flow workout. If you are looking to achieve greater flexibility while embracing the concept of softness is strength, Sadhana Yoga definitely answers this call.

Softness Is Power

There are two diametrically opposite concepts for embracing a powerful physical work-out: you can either deplete your powerful energy during your workout and end up being tired, or enhance your energy while practicing your yoga and find yourself refreshed afterward. When you complete a strenuous workout like kickboxing, soccer, or high-impact aerobic dance, you are actually depleting your energy and going against the natural flow. Through the quest to get a good workout, most people expend more energy than they consume oxygen. Also there is a lot of wasted and unfocused energy. The same holds true in yoga practice. If you move too fast, don't focus on your deep breathing, and waste a lot of strength unnecessarily or you will feel a loss of your potential energy.

Yoga is not meant to be practiced the way most people practice sports. Sadhana Yoga is designed to enhance your energy, not deplete it. When you focus on your deep breathing, surrender to the posture, take your time and build energy during your workout, you will automatically go with the natural flow of energy. You are instead conserving your energy by moving softly, quietly, and yet with the power of that beautiful river.

In Sadhana Yoga you will learn to go with the natural lines of energy, rather than fighting against them. The natural lines of energy is the organic flow of energy which creates the least resistance or stress, and can be effected by internal and external forces. To go with the flow of energy, you will be surrendering to the posture. You will learn not to fight against your yoga practice. For example, if you are doing a Downward Facing Dog Posture you can fight against the pull of Earth by holding your back high, or relax and allow the gravity to gently lengthen your neck and upper back in a more neutral posture and allow the energy from Earth to run through your body. In this manor you learn to use the power of the whole universe to work with you rather than against you.

Gaining Flexibility with Sadhana Yoga

Flexibility is attained through the stretching and lengthening of your muscles. There are other types of exercise which have various different stretching techniques, yet they all stem from traditional yoga.

Gaining flexibility is one of the reasons that originally made yoga so very popular. The Sadhana Yoga program will gradually touch every aspect of flexibility. My program is designed to accommodate all levels of practice, from the stiff occasional weekend stretcher to the real Gumby, or advanced yoga student. The stretching component of this program can be divided into three categories: warm-up *asanas*, traditional yoga postures and their counter stretching, and *vinyasas*, or linking stretches.

Warm-up *asanas* are yoga exercises designed to increase your circulation, thereby creating more internal heat and making your muscles more pliable before beginning the yoga postures themselves. Yoga warm-up exercises also create a tranquil mood; this will help to transcend your mind into the practice. Yoga warm-ups are movement exercises, as opposed to the traditional yoga postures, which are considered to be stationary postures.

In Sadhana Yoga I divide the traditional yoga postures into eight different categories: seated postures, inversions, leg stretches, back stretches, twisting exercises, arm-strengthening stretches, standing balance stretches, and relaxation postures. Each of these stretches are balanced with counter-stretches, which stretch your body in the opposite direction, balancing the body back to its natural state after completing a stretch. In the Sadhana Yoga program counter stretches are incorporated into the routine, with complete instructions as to how you might add additional counter stretches as you see fit. For example, if you have practiced numerous back-stretching postures, you may want to add a Forward Bend as a counter stretch to balance out your muscles.

Vinyasa stretching is the stretching you receive as you practice the flowing-link movements from one yoga posture to the next. A *vinyasa* is basically a continuous flow of stretching and counter stretching created to transport you to another posture, while creating heat and embracing the natural energy flow. If you were to stop the movement of your *vinyasa* in the middle, you might find your *vinyasa* stretching looking like a typical yoga posture.

Increasing Endurance Through Sadhana Yoga

Endurance factors are directly related to your heart strength, working in combination with your muscles and lungs. Endurance relates to the amount of time you remain within a sustained physical activity. If you can only maintain your physical activity for a short amount of time, then your endurance factor is low. If you can maintain a physical activity for a long period of time, then your endurance factor is high.

You can increase your endurance qualities through gradually practicing longer physical workouts with periods of rest in between. In time you will take fewer rests and develop a more sustained workout. Another way to increase you endurance is by holding each of your yoga postures for longer durations. Over a period of weeks or months you can start adding more physically challenging yoga postures to your routine, as you build more strength. In the long run you will create a more physical practice and be able to maintain this for longer periods of time.

In order to encompass the full balanced spectrum of Sadhana Yoga, it is best to practice Soft-Flow workouts one day and more physical routines the next. You are in effect cross-training between the Hard- and Soft-Flow workouts.

Developing the Mind Flow

Very few of us function with our body and mind in unison. If you can totally connect your thoughts with your actions, the results are quite amazing. In sports, dance, martial arts, or leisure activities, a mind-body connection can mean the difference between falling on your face or smoothly gliding with grace and elegance.

One of the main goals of yoga is in the unification of mind-body action. You have to master your mind before you can master your body. Whether you choose to follow a Hard- or Soft-Flow workout, you also need to develop your yoga practice from within. Your beautifully flowing, yet powerfully physical yoga practice mirrors your beautiful, yet powerful mind and inward energy. During Sadhana Yoga, this powerful mind element is connected at all times to the body, yet remains focused and calm. Your thoughts are in the moment, not scattered dealing with other worldly issues. Only when the two aspects of mind and body are working together can true harmony and grace be achieved.

To develop this mind flow and realize this wonderful yoga practice, you need to harness a variety of internal tools: *bandhas*, breathing, and *drishti.* By using these three wonderful tools you will conscientiously use your mind to create inner harmony and greater focus. This will then affect your yoga posture practice, increasing your vital life force energy, or *prana.*

Bandhas: *The Gateways of Internal Power*

The first natural tool your mind can make use of during yoga practice is the *bandha*, or energy lock. You engage a *bandha* through the concentrated effort of contracting certain muscles within your body. These contractions or locks direct the flow of *prana* energy you create during yoga practice, also helping to create stability and inward strength. *Bandhas* give your mind and your entire body an energy lift during your *vinyasas*, added control during your *asanas*, as well as toning up your stomach and internal organs. By engaging your *bandhas*, you maintain greater control and focus over your body's actions, which lead to the knowledge that you can control and focus your mind as well. *Bandhas* are actually muscle groups and pressure points within your body. Each of the three primary *bandhas* has its own name:

I. *Mula bandha*: The *mula bandha* is called the root lock, and is located in the perineal muscles between your genitals and anus. To engage these muscles, imagine that you are in a car and find yourself having to go to the bathroom, and the nearest one is five miles away. As you take that long journey, you engage your *mula bandha* in order to avoid an unfortunate accident. In yoga practice, you will engage your *mula bandha* through the lifting and contracting of the perineal muscles.

2. *Uddiyana bandha:* The name *uddiyana* translates as meaning "flying up." This *bandha* is located about three fingers below your navel. To engage this *bandha* you focus on your lower abdominal muscles as you lift them slightly and contract your stomach, which then draws up your diaphragm. During yoga practice you always use the *uddiyana bandha* in conjunction with *mula bandha* to give you strength and stability while firming your abdominal muscles and help you embrace greater *prana* energy.

3. *Jalandhara bandha:* The *jalandhara bandha* is called the "chin lock." You engage this *bandha* by stretching the back of the neck as you lower your chin into the notch in your breastbone. This *bandha* is used in a few postures like the Shoulder Stand and Staff postures, yet more frequently in some *pranayama* breathing exercises. You will not use *jalandhara bandha* nearly as often as you use the *mula bandha* or the *uddiyana bandha*.

Using Bandhas to Enhance Your Practice

To get the most out of your practice, you should engage your *mula* and *uddiyana bandhas* each time that you are holding a yoga posture. You should then release the *bandha* as you leave a posture. You will reengage the *bandhas* during your *vinyasa* linking movements: they will give you extra strength when the *vinyasa* involves lifting your body weight.

Yoga Breathing Made Simple

The Sanskrit word *pranayama* is attributed to the science and practice of breath control. It is a combination of two important terms, *prana*, which is the vital life force, and *yama*, which means "discipline." *Prana* represents all of the elements of life: earth, air, fire, water, and ether. Yoga practice helps you extract these elements from nature through controlled breathing, which replenishes the pranic energy. Taking this concept one step further, many great yoga masters have expressed the idea that air is a food. They believe that if you cleanse the body of toxins and live in a clean, fresh environment, then air can serve as a supplemental nutritional source. The best, highly energy-charged air is available near mountains, waterfalls, and oceans, all areas abundant with negatively charged ions. I can tell you from experience that when I practice yoga in areas where you have a good supply of negatively charged ions, it is an incredibly powerful experience.

In our daily lives, most of us tend to take very shallow breaths. Over time this incomplete breathing can reduce your overall health and vitality. Yoga breathing is quite different from regular breathing. By consciously making an effort to maintain correct breathing, we are rewarded with more energy, less stress, and better mental focus. With each breath you will better oxygenate your blood and muscles, and supply fresh oxygen to your brain. You will be expanding your lungs, greatly increasing their capacity and ability to fuel your body. What's more, the slow and deep breathing rhythm in Sadhana Yoga creates more energy, and at the same time generates a calm, yet focused mind during both Hard- and Soft-Flow practice, as well as in your everyday life.

Yoga breathing has three distinct qualities:

1. **The complete breath:** For each breath you take, you completely fill your lungs with air on inhalation *(puraka)* and completely empty your lungs on exhalation *(rechaka)*. Holding your breath is called *kumbaka*.

2. **Slow deep breathing:** In Sadhana Yoga, your breathing is slow, steady, deep, and rhythmic. This controlled breathing enables you to take more oxygen into your lungs, leaving you feeling refreshed and invigorated after practice. It also creates a calm and relaxed mind.

3. **Sound breathing (*ujjayi*):** The specific technique of yoga breathing is called *ujjayi*, which translates as meaning "victorious breath." It involves inhaling and exhaling air through your nose. As you breathe in through your nose, the incoming air makes a soft, hissing sound on the back of your throat. This tranquil, meditative sound, in combination with your slow, deep, and calculated breathing pattern, contributes to enhancing your energy, calming of your body and mind, and enabling you to center your thoughts on your practice.

INSTRUCTIONS FOR *UJJAYI* BREATHING:

1. Sit comfortably on the floor or in a chair with a straight back. Place your hands loosely at your sides.

2. Engage your *bandhas* by keeping your abdominal muscles firm and slightly contracted. Close your eyes and take a slow, deep breath through your nose. Inhale fully until your lungs feel completely expanded and your rib cage feels lifted.

3. Slowly exhale through your nose. As you exhale, your chest sinks and your lungs contract. Your abdominal muscles remain slightly engaged throughout the breathing cycle. This does not mean you should stress or force your abdominal muscles not to expand. A little expansion is normal, yet you should strive toward expanding your chest and not your belly.

4. Try it again, but this time as you inhale, slightly restrict, or squeeze the air with your throat muscles. Now, exhale through your nose as you once again slightly restrict the air flow by squeezing the air with your throat muscles. Try one more time, this time without tensing, just relax, and on the inhalation, think of drawing energy into your body. Then exhale through your nose, with the same technique as the inhalation, only now think of releasing stress and tension. This time you will notice that you are making a strong hissing sound through your nose.

5. Continue with your breathing slowly, deeply, and controlled. With each inhalation and exhalation, slightly tighten your throat muscles as you feel and hear the air swirling past your throat.

Sadhana Yoga Breathing vs. Traditional Yoga Breathing

While all forms of yoga breathing are similar, each has its own subtle yet important differences. In traditional soft-style yoga, many teachers use a similar *ujjayi* breathing technique you have just learned in this section, although in some traditional yoga breathing, you are often taught to expand the lower abdominal muscles on inhalations and contract the lower abdominal muscles on the exhalation. In Sadhana Yoga you will keep these muscles firm in order to assist in creating core strength and control.

In some powerful forms of yoga practice the breath is often a bit rushed, which can lead to a loss of potential energy and sacrifice the tranquil yoga flow. Within Sadhana Yoga you are encouraged to adapt a continuous slow, deep breathing rhythm to enhance energy, as well as creating inner calm and focus. Other styles of yoga practice do not embrace breathing as an important point within the practice, which will only limit the energy potential. In Sadhana Yoga the breathing is the strong foundation on which to build a successful practice.

Pranayama *Breathing Exercises*

The following two breathing techniques are categorized as *pranayama*. Simply by learning to control your breathing techniques, you can feed you heart and brain, create heat and energy, or cool yourself down to relax, releasing stress, and create a very soothing touch throughout your whole body. As you inhale you will increase the vital life-force energy, and as you exhale you will release toxins, stress, and tension to create deep relaxation, inward harmony, and greater focus.

EXERCISE #1: BELLOWS BREATHING

In this exercise your breathing will simulate a tool called a bellows, which was often used to blow more oxygen into a flame, thereby increasing the fire and allowing it to burn more efficiently. When you practice Bellows Breathing you will stoke your internal flame and create more energy. This exercise can be used after yoga practice in order to help replenish your vital life-force energy. The immediate effect is one of energy, and this moves into a very calm and relaxed state of being.

INSTRUCTIONS

1. Sit on the floor with your arms extended out over your knees, with your hands resting on your knees, palms facing downward. If you find it more comfortable, you may elevate your hips by sitting on the edge of a small pillow or blanket. If your hips are very stiff, you may also place small pillows up under your knees. You can also choose to sit on the edge of a chair with your hands resting on your thighs (palms facing downward) and your feet resting on the floor, about six inches apart.

2. Embrace good posture with your spine straight and shoulders back; imagine a thin beam of golden light coming into the top of your head lifting you upward to create better alignment.

3. Sit calm and relax for a few seconds as you embrace the slow deep yoga breathing, completely filling your lungs with air on inhalations and completely emptying your lungs on exhalations.

4. Now proceed into the Bellows Breathing. You will inhale and exhale through your nose, with very short and quick repetitions, lift your shoulders and ribs on inhalations, and collapse then on exhalations. One inhalation and one exhalation equals one round, repeat this exercise for 10 to 20 rounds, then relax into your regular, slow, deep yoga breathing for a few more breaths, as you sit quietly and relax.

EXERCISE #2: ALTERNATE BREATHING

This exercise will assist with opening the sinuses, releasing body toxins, creating more energy, and at the same time embracing a feeling of complete relaxation and peace of mind. Practice this wonderful breathing exercise by itself, after your yoga practice, or right before deep relaxation.

Hand placement for Alternate Breathing—Using your right hand, allow your first two fingertips to bend in and touch the middle of your thumb. Let your hand muscles stay relaxed, as you use the thumb to seal off your right nostril and your ring and little finger to seal off your left nostril.

1. Choose one of your favorite seated postures and sit quietly while practicing five slow deep breaths with complete inhalations and complete exhalations. Allow your arms to extend out over your knees, with the palms of your hands facing upward and fingers placed in *Jnana Mudra* (see page 52).

2. Exhale all your air completely, then seal off your right nostril with your right thumb, completely filling your lungs through your left nostril.

3. Seal off both nostrils, holding your breath and engaging all three *bandhas*. Hold for about 15 seconds, then seal off your left nostril with your ring and little fingers and exhale through your right nostril as you release your *bandhas*.

4. Inhale again through your right nostril and seal off both nostrils and hold your breath for another 15 seconds. Then seal off your right nostril and exhale out your left nostril. This is one round. Complete three rounds, then relax, sit quietly, and take five complete yoga breaths through both nostrils.

In this posture you will resemble a lion as it roars. This breathing exercise relaxes facial muscles, and helps to expel smoke and pollution from your lungs. It can also help to relieve a sore throat.

INSTRUCTIONS

1. Start by sitting on the floor, resting on your knees, as you sit on top of your heels. Sit upright with good posture. Rest your hands on your knees with palms facing downward.

2. Inhale, completely filling your lungs with air, then exhale forcefully through your mouth, pushing the air out with your abdominal muscles. At the same time open your mouth wide, stick your tongue out, and exhale as you make a sound of "HAAA." This simulates the roar of a lion.

3. Stretch your fingers out like lion claws on the exhalation. Practice three rounds, then sit calmly and relax for a few breaths.

Drishti: *Focusing on the Internal Gaze*

In some yoga styles, much emphasis is placed on the way you direct and hold your gaze during practice. These fixed points are assigned for each posture and are called the *drishti*. The word *drishti* means both "looking out" and "looking in."

The purpose of the *drishti* is not to get your vision fixed on a particular place or part of your body; it's actually an exercise to help you turn your gaze inward, so that you can place your attention on your *bandhas,* breathing, and posture alignment. Gazing inward is considered to be a form of sense withdrawal; the *drishti* is then a tool to help you in this part of yoga practice. When you "use the *drishti*," you are more focused on your internal yoga, and less apt to be distracted by external actions. This gaze has an impact on your physical and mental state during each posture, and your ability to remain focused and energized.

In Sadhana Yoga, students are taught to gaze into a posture's "stretch." This means to gaze in the direction of your stretch in any given posture and then turn your focus inward. Students are also encouraged to focus on the line of least resistance, which can be an individualized aspect. For example, if you are very flexible and practicing a Seated Forward Bend, gazing at your toes will create tension in your neck. In this case you would lower your vision toward your legs. On the other hand, less flexible people will find least resistance by gazing at their toes. Personally, I prefer not to be too strict with the *drishti*, and have found through experience the aspect of gazing in the direction of the stretch and the individualized approach of gazing along the lines of least resistance to be most useful.

BEING MINDFUL OF THE MOMENT

You can accomplish a lot more in your life, and your yoga practice, by being present in the moment, totally aware of all that is going on around you, in control and at peace. If you always think of how things will get better later, or how you will relax and do what you want later, later may never arrive. In your yoga practice you should enjoy this special and sacred moment as a precious gift. Be in the moment; experience the struggle as much as the blissful relaxation. Live your life for today and tomorrow will wait for you.

YOGA POSTURES AND FLOWING LINKS

Beauty is yoga

Flowing effortless

With strength and grace

Yoga postures are the various postures held for specific amounts of time. In Sanskrit these yoga postures are called *asanas,* which means "posture comfortably held." The yoga postures in Sadhana Yoga form the base of your program and act as a positive influence, or catalyst, for every other aspect of your life. The flowing links refer to the movements between the yoga postures, or the specific manner in which you enter and exit each posture. In Sanskrit this movement is called *vinyasa.*

The philosophy of Sadhana Yoga is more than just stretching in yoga postures and breathing; it is a method to connect your body and mind with the energy of the whole universe. Sadhana Yoga is also about learning to channel the energy from the Earth and into your practice.

Knowing When to Practice

Before you actually begin your journey of yoga practice, there are a few things you need to think about. Yoga at any time of day is a wonderful gift, as your body and mind will surely thank you for the experience. However, the best times of the day to practice, should you be fortunate enough, is at sunrise and sunset. At sunrise and sunset the energy of the sun is either just starting up or just closing down. These transitional time periods create a tranquil atmosphere, which is very conducive to yoga practice.

BEFORE OR AFTER OTHER EXERCISE?

Yoga is a very complete system, yet other physical activities will serve to enhance your yoga, and your yoga will enhance your other physical activities. If you plan on engaging in other strenuous activities on the same day that you do your yoga practice, try to do those other activities first, and end with your yoga practice. Yoga is a very balanced system, which will correct your body alignment, soothe your muscles, and relax your mind. If you can schedule yoga after your other strenuous activities, the benefits of your practice will stay with you much longer. Light or moderate physical activities can be done either before or after yoga practice.

Eating and Yoga Practice

Ideally, you should begin yoga practice on an empty stomach, or one hour after eating a moderate meal, and two hours after eating a large meal. It is very important not to eat a heavy meal right before you plan on doing your yoga. Eating right before yoga will make you uncomfortable, less flexible, and disrupt the energy flow. If you must have something before practice, try drinking fresh squeezed juice, a smoothie, or eat a light meal of fruits or vegetables. Try fresh-squeezed green vegetable juice, mixed with a little carrot or apple; this will supply you with natural energy for hours and takes only minutes to digest.

Where to Practice

It is not always possible to have the ideal location to practice in, so do the best you can with what you have. Whether you are at home or in a yoga studio or on a mountaintop, make sure that you are in an area with a comfortable temperature which is neither too hot or too cold. Your practice should ideally be conducted in a moderate to slightly warm temperature. If it is too cold, you will not be as flexible and have greater chance of injury. If it is too hot, you will drain your energy and dehydrate. If you find that your only option is to practice in a cold location, wear more layers of clothing.

> *Outdoor vs. Indoor*—The perfect temperature for outdoor yoga is anywhere between 70 and 100 degrees Fahrenheit. Try to avoid practicing in the noonday sun: moderate sun exposure is healthy in early morning and late evening.

If you are practicing indoors, make sure that there are plenty of plants in the room and that the room has good ventilation. Plants give off oxygen and filter pollution! If you fill an enclosed room full of people exercising and doing deep breathing without plants, they will use up all the fresh air, creating an atmosphere of oxygen deprivation. This quality of air is worse than on pollution-alert days. Remember, yoga enhances your *prana* through breath, and if there is no fresh air in the room, then you are greatly restricting your benefits.

Moderate artificial heat is fine as long as the room is not too hot. A yoga room should be heated to around 80 degrees. If the room is heated over 80 degrees, the heat can make your heart work harder, disrupting the energy flow and causing excessive dehydration. Ideally, through your yoga practice you will learn to generate your own heat from within.

> *Pleasing atmosphere*—Choose a comfortable, relaxing, and clean environment free from annoying noise, paint fumes, and any other major distractions. You may want to play light background music, or just listen to your own breath and practice. Also, if you create an indoor environment which is pleasing to your eye, this will help set a better mood for practice.

Practicing Alone or in a Group?

Ideally you should find some time to practice alone on one day and next time in a group. The following session practice with a friend. Practicing alone is a great way to find your innermost qualities in a noncompetitive atmosphere. Practicing with a friend can be very rewarding and helpful with assistance in your individual yoga postures. It is very nice to share the sacred practice of yoga. Help each other, or just practice together and be silent. Practicing in a group has the advantage of group energy, quality instruction, and the social aspects of being around like-minded people.

Choosing an Instructor

Probably the most important decision you have to make when beginning to practice yoga is finding an instructor who will help you along your path. Unfortunately, due to the popularity of yoga, there are many unqualified instructors who are now "certified" to teach. Never judge a teacher's qualifications solely by a piece of paper: always ask how long it took them to get their certification and how many years they have been practicing and teaching. If you look for yoga certification, make sure that the yoga instructor you choose is certified and registered through the national Yoga Alliance.

Aside from certification, choose yoga teachers who have at least several years of experience and are kind, compassionate, self-confident, willing to work with your own needs, and practice what they preach. Just because a teacher has had lots of local press, is very popular, or appears on the cover of a yoga magazine does not make them the best teacher. Remember, no one instructor or *guru* has all the answers, although they might make that claim. A very wise sage once said, "All ways are right and one way is wrong." Find a teacher you enjoy, yet also study from a variety of different teachers as well in order to build a more complete practice.

Learning How to Practice

In your yoga practice take your time, move slowly, and be kind to yourself. Pick a yoga routine within your own spectrum of practice: working over your head is very discouraging and often uncomfortable. Yoga practice should be approached as something very sacred and valuable. This does not mean you have to lose your sense of humor. After all, laughter is the best medicine and you should enjoy your practice. Yoga deserves the same consideration and attention you would give to a true love. Be kind, loving, and gentle, move with softness and grace from one posture to the next.

Hints and Cautions

Yoga is a wonderful system of movement and can greatly affect your whole physical and mental outlook in a positive way. However, injuries can occur. Always listen to your body. A little pain is good, yet consistent pain for weeks in a row is a sign of neglect. Knowing your limits is the sign of a true *yogi* or *yogini*. As an advanced student, you should take it easy now and then and cross-train with other activities to help avoid and overcome injury.

Whether you are a student or a teacher, it is always good to ask questions when you are unsure about a yoga posture. Most important, let your yoga evolve slowly, and try not to be competitive: you can progress quicker simply by challenging yourself, not others. Everyone who practices yoga is a winner, not just the ones who stretch and bend farther.

Moving with Grace

Time and experience teaches you to go with the flow of your practice. Your practice should become very smooth and fluid and, ultimately, take on the quality of a slow, soft dance. As you combine these gentle yet powerful movements with your deep breathing and mental focus, you gain the maximum benefit.

When you are transitioning from one posture to the next, try to enter and exit each posture with grace and elegance. When I first learned yoga, I moved between the postures like a clumsy, raging bull. As I refined my technique I came to think of each posture as a delicate flower. As I moved between them, I tried to float like a butterfly, so as not to disturb the calm beauty of the posture once I "landed."

In the unique system of Sadhana Yoga, you develop power by developing softness. The more controlled, smooth, and gentle your movements, the more they strengthen your body. And the way you move has a large impact on your state of mind. When your body is jumping and jerking, your mind is less focused and unsettled. But when you float with the power of the wind, your mind is calm, relaxed, focused, and in control.

Props and Tools

Props are tools that make yoga practice a bit easier for the uninitiated beginner, especially if you have special physical needs, such as recovering from an injury. The use of props can greatly assist in comfort and alignment, and lay the groundwork for you to achieve the posture on your own. If you think that you can benefit from props, then by all means use them. Try not to be totally dependant on them, so that they keep you from improving.

Here are some of the more popular props:

Yoga practice mats—Used to create better traction, warmth, and comfort. They are generally made of a sticky rubber. There are nonsticky mats made from cotton material.

Straps—Yoga straps have many uses such as to assist in extending your reach, correcting alignment, and enabling partner work. Try straps to assist in Seated Forward Bends.

Blocks—Very helpful in assisting with balance, extending your reach, creating torso lift, and great for *vinyasa* Jump Throughs.

Wedges—Can be used to help overcome wrist problems and to give assistance with tight leg muscles in Downward Facing Dog.

Eye pillows—Are a great way to help you melt into deep relaxation, blocking out light and soothing your eyes.

Towels—Are nice especially if you are in a hot and physical class. You can use towels as a tool to extend your reach, or as a prop to lift your hips during seated postures.

A bottle of water—is a great idea; you can never be too hydrated.

BEGIN WITH BREATHING

You are now ready to begin Sadhana Yoga practice. Read through the rest of the chapter before beginning any postures. The first step is to get your breathing under control. Refer back to Chapter 3 to understand the breathing techniques more fully.

As you move through your Sadhana Yoga routines, remember to move in sync with your yoga breathing techniques. You can use your breathing to assist in the energy flow from which you move from one yoga posture to the next. Here are a few basic guidelines for coordinating your breathing and movement during *vinyasa* practice:

1. Exhale and relax as you move into any yoga posture, and inhale, creating strength, as you move out.

2. Inhale when you are going against gravity, and exhale when you are going with gravity.

3. Inhale before you move into a strength *vinyasa*, and then relax into the movement.

4. On inhalations embrace strength and energy from the Earth, and on exhalations release stress and tension creating softness and tranquility.

LEARNING THE *ASANA* POSTURES

The goal of yoga posture practice is to find balance and create harmony physically, mentally, and spirituality by finding balance between your strength and softness. The postures should be respected and treated as a sacred spiritual creation, not just another type of physical fitness. Yoga postures can be divided into nine categories, each affecting a separate area or aspect of your body.

Yoga Sequencing

When creating a yoga routine, the aspect of yoga sequencing should not be overlooked, or you will risk injury, lose energy, and disrupt the flow. In the categories listed below, I have arranged the categories in proper sequence. If you are creating your own routine, simply start at the first category and progress toward the end, picking one or two postures from each category.

Categories of Yoga Postures

1. **Seated postures:** These are some of the most fundamental aspects of yoga practice. They give you a good base for practicing breathing exercises and meditation, and act as a transition for moving into, or out of, a practice routine. Just as yoga breathing isn't the same as normal breathing, sitting during yoga isn't the same old thing you do every day. You don't want to just dash into the seated postures like a winner on a television game show. In order to get the most from your whole routine, you need to enter the seated postures slowly, embracing correct body alignment and breathing techniques.

2. **Warm-ups:** Every yoga routine begins with traditional warm-up exercises. These will increase your circulation, warm your muscles, and at the same time give you a chance to connect with a natural flowing movement of energy.

Warm-up exercises and traditional yoga postures are similar, yet different. Yoga warm-ups are designed to create internal heat, start the *prana* energy flowing, and get your whole body prepared for the postures themselves. On the other hand, yoga postures follow a definite sequence, are held for a specific amount of time, and are usually connected with specific anatomical benefits.

3. **Inverted postures and counter stretches:** Inverted postures refers to postures which place your body upside down and affect your whole body, creating a passive and calm state of mind, yet leaving you very refreshed and rejuvenated. After you spend many hours each day with your body in an upright position, inverted postures can reverse any negative effects. The most popular inverted yoga postures are the Headstand and Shoulder Stand.

Caution: Inverted postures should be avoided if you have any of the following physical conditions:

- *a floating retina*
- *during your menstrual cycle*
- *severe injury to your neck*
- *glaucoma*
- *extreme high blood pressure*

Counter Stretching refers to the experience of stretching one side of your body after completing a series of stretches on the opposite side. For example, if you completed a back bend and find tension in your back, you could add a counter stretch such as a Seated Forward Bend to release the tension and return your body to a neutral state.

4. **Leg stretches:** Leg stretch postures lengthen and tone your leg muscles, joints, and tendons. These postures will create more pliable muscles, release stress and tension, and help to prepare you for many other postures.

5. **Back-bending postures:** Back-bending postures focus on arching your back. They lengthen, tone, and stretch your spine. These postures will create a more pliable spine and help to assist in proper vertebrae alignment. In addition, these postures help to expand your chest, correct round shoulders, and strengthen back muscles. Keep your back healthy and strong through regular moderate yoga exercise, and you will be active throughout your life.

6. **Twisting postures:** Twisting postures focus on your spine and back muscles by twisting, toning, and stretching your spine. These postures will create a more pliable spine and help to assist in proper vertebrae alignment. In addition these postures help to overcome backaches and create more mobility of your spine and whole torso.

7. **Arm-balance postures:** Arm-balance postures strengthen your arms, shoulders, and upper body. These postures also create self-confidence, enhance balance, and teach the philosophy that softness is power. Arm-balance postures will create muscle strength and toning by lifting your own body weight. Generally speaking, these postures tend to be easier for intermediate to advanced students, although beginners should still give them a try.

8. **Standing postures:** Standing postures are achieved by standing on one or both feet. They can strengthen your legs, creating balance and self-confidence.

9. **Deep relaxation postures:** Relaxation postures are used at the end of yoga practice, or during relaxation and meditation exercises. They are designed to embrace a very relaxing element where you can embrace positive thinking and peace of mind.

THE YOGA POSTURES

CATEGORY #1: SEATED POSTURES—

Handling Your Hands With Jnana Mudra—*(All levels)*

In Sanskrit, *jnana* means "knowledge" and a *mudra* means "seal" or "lock." Often seated postures include specific placement of your hands and fingers. Traditionally, yogis use *Jnana Mudra* as they meditate. In *Jnana Mudra*, your index finger represents your individual soul, and your thumb represents the universal soul. As you unite the tip of your thumb to the tip of your index finger, you symbolically unite the energy of your soul with the energy of the whole universe. The result of this unification is knowledge.

1. Sit on the floor in any of your favorite seated postures listed in this section.

2. Place your hands on your knees with your palms facing upward.

3. Open your hands and touch your index finger to the tip of your thumb. Your remaining fingers should be straight, but not stiff or tense.

The Seated Angle Posture—Upavistha Konasana *(All levels)*

The Seated Angle is a base to enter and exit many postures and *vinyasas*. You can use this posture for meditation practice as well.

BENEFITS

The Seated Angle Posture corrects your posture, strengthens the muscles of your back, and opens the energy flow in your chest. Many people who have trouble with their knees will find the Seated Angle a good alternative to the cross-legged seated postures.

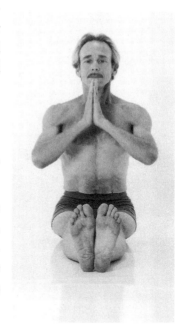

INSTRUCTIONS

1. Sit on the floor with both legs extended out in front, your spine straight, and your shoulders back.

2. Keep your feet pointing upward and slightly flexed, as you place your hands in prayer fashion over your chest. If your lower back is rounded, try placing a small pillow under your knees: this can help nudge your body into the proper posture. Hold this posture for five to ten slow, deep breaths.

Perfect Posture—Siddhasana *(All levels)*

In Sanskrit, *siddha* means "perfect." A *siddha* is also a great prophet or a sage, one who is very pure and spiritual. As you practice Perfect Posture, you're connecting with the wisdom of the ancient yoga masters.

Perfect Posture promotes flexibility in your knees, ankles, and thighs, and it also contributes to attaining excellent posture.

INSTRUCTIONS

1. Start by sitting on the floor with your legs extended out in front of you, with your spine straight and your shoulders back in the Seated Angle Posture listed above.

2. Bend your right knee, grabbing your right ankle with your hands and pulling your foot in toward your groin. Now grab your left ankle and pull your left foot in toward your groin, placing your left foot under your right knee.

3. Now you are sitting cross-legged on the floor with your spine straight and your shoulders back in Perfect Posture. If you find this uncomfortable, place a small pillow under each knee. In addition you might choose to place a small pillow under you hips in order to help correct your posture. More flexible students can lower their knees to the floor. For **beginners**, as an alternative you could sit on the edge of the chair, keeping your back straight with feet flat on the floor and hands in your lap.

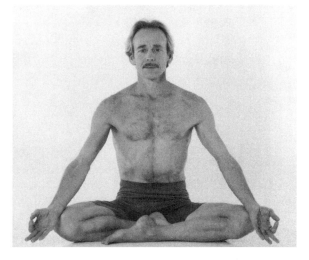

4. Extend your arms and rest your wrists and hands on your knees, with palms facing upward. Now place your fingers in the traditional *Jnana Mudra* Position. Hold this posture for five to ten slow, deep yoga breaths, calm your mind, and relax.

Full Lotus—Padmasana *(Intermediate to Advanced)*

The word *padma* means "lotus." In this posture, you float like a water lily as you create the beauty of a lotus flower with your body and your mind. This is a very advanced posture, so be extremely gentle with your knees, and take your time.

BENEFITS

This posture helps invigorate the nerves in your legs and thighs. It also helps loosen your knee joints, increases flexibility in your ankles, and opens hips.

INSTRUCTIONS

1. Sit on the floor in Perfect Posture as listed above, with your back straight, your mind calm. You should be completely focused and relaxed.

2. Take your left foot in your hands and slowly place it on your right thigh.

3. Take your right foot in your hands and slowly place it on your left thigh.

4. Be aware of correct posture as you open your chest and gently pull your shoulders back. Feel yourself relax as you sit proudly with your chin held high.

5. Extend your arms over your thighs and rest your hands and wrists on your knees, with palms facing upward.

6. Place your hands in *Jnana Mudra*. You now are in the Full Lotus Posture.

7. Close your eyes and hold this posture for five to ten slow deep breaths, calm the mind and relax, as you feel yourself gently floating. Try to practice engaging the *mula* and *uddiyana bandhas*.

8. When you are finished, open your eyes, grab your right ankle with your hands, and slowly lower your right foot back to the floor and take hold of your left ankle with your right hand, lowering your left ankle to the floor.

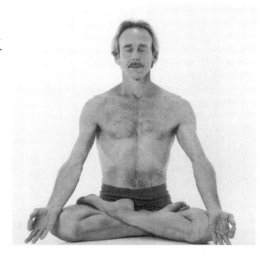

In order to keep a balance of stretch, the next time you practice Lotus Posture, place your right foot up on your left thigh first.

Bound Lotus (Baddha Padmasana)—(Advanced)

The word *baddha* means "caught or restrained" and *padmasana* is the Lotus Posture. In this posture you will restrain your feet with your hands and arms.

BENEFITS

In this posture you will receive the same benefits as the Lotus, plus an extra stretch through your arms, shoulders, and chest.

INSTRUCTIONS

1. Start from the Full Lotus Posture, reach behind your back with your left hand and grab the toes of your left foot. If necessary, lean forward until you can take hold of your toes.

2. Repeat this process to reach behind your back with your right hand to grab toes of your right foot.

3. Sit up gradually, maintaining correct posture. Close your eyes, relax, and hold this posture for five to fifteen slow deep breaths.

4. When you are finished, open your eyes and release the grip of your hands on your toes. Take your feet out of lotus slowly and stretch your legs out straight for a few breaths.

Thunderbolt (Vajrasana)—(All levels)

The Sanskrit word *vajra* means thunderbolt. Sometimes this same posture is referred to as either Hero or Champion. This posture is a good alternative for the cross-legged postures, and is commonly used as a base posture for meditation.

BENEFITS

The Thunderbolt stimulates the nerves in your feet and lower legs, and stretches the muscles in your feet and ankles. In fact, many yoga masters use this posture to correct flat feet and promote better arches. It also creates more flexibility in your knees and can help improve your posture.

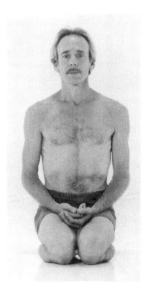

INSTRUCTIONS

1. Kneel on the floor, keeping your spine straight and shoulders back.

2. Sit back on your heels with your toes pointed backward. Feel your neck lengthen, and then fold your hands into your lap. Another variation which is especially helpful when your have knee problems is to place a rolled up towel or small pillow between your calves and thighs.

4. Place your gaze straight head, parallel to the floor. Hold Thunderbolt Posture for five to ten complete breaths.

Child's Posture—(Balasana)—(All levels)

The word *Bala* refers to a child, and in this posture you will resemble a young child stretching on the floor. The Child's Posture is used as a great relaxation posture in itself, or as a counter stretch for Headstand, and other back-bending postures.

BENEFITS

In the Child's Posture you will create a soothing lengthening effect on your vertebrae and stretch tension out of your arms, shoulders, and back.

INSTRUCTIONS

1. Start from the Thunderbolt Posture listed above. Extend your arms forward onto the floor above your head, with your forehead 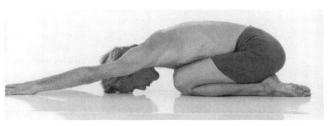 resting on the floor. If you have tight hips and legs, place a small pillow up under your hips and another up under your torso for support.

2. Hold this position for five complete breaths. When finished, inhale and return to the Thunderbolt Posture and relax.

Neck Rolls—(All levels)

Neck rolls are exactly what their name implies. In this exercise you will gently roll and stretch your neck. Make sure to move slowly and practice your yoga breathing throughout the exercise.

BENEFITS

Neck rolls serve to warm up the muscles of your neck, release tension, and create flexibility.

INSTRUCTIONS

1. To begin, choose one of the seated postures, or sit on the edge of a chair. Sit up straight with good posture as you maintain slow deep breathing throughout the exercise.

2. Start by tilting your head slowly, moving it gently forward and backward. Now tilt your head slowly from side to side, keeping your vision forward, as if you were going to touch your ear to your shoulder. First tilt your head slowly and gently to the right side, and then back to the left side.

3. Now turn your head to the right, looking over your right shoulder. Return to facing forward, and repeat by turning your head to the left, looking back over your left shoulder. Repeat this left and right motion two times.

4. Proceed to roll your neck slowly and gently in a circular motion first to the right two times, and then back to the left two times. Be careful when tilting your head backward: and if you feel an area with a kink, or pulled muscle, just go around that spot. When finished, just sit quietly and breathe for a few breaths.

Shoulder Rolls—(All levels)

Shoulder rolls get their name from the rolling motion of your shoulders. Make sure to move slowly and practice your yoga breathing throughout the exercise.

BENEFITS

Shoulder Rolls serve to warm up the muscles of your shoulders and upper back, release tension, and create a bit of flexibility.

INSTRUCTIONS

1. To begin, choose one of the seated postures, or sit on the edge of a chair. Sit up straight with good posture, as you maintain slow deep breathing throughout the exercise.

2. Start by lifting your shoulders up by your ears, and then rotate your shoulders back behind your head. Complete the circle by lowering your shoulders downward and then forward.

3. Strive to make this exercise flow in a circular motion, first in one direction for a few repetitions, then change directions and roll your shoulders back in the other direction.

4. When finished, sit quietly and relax for a few breaths.

Eagle Wings—(All levels)

In this exercise you will resemble an eagle as it stretches its wings before flight. This warm-up movement can also be used as a subtle *vinyasa* for energy postures.

BENEFITS

Eagle Wings helps to release tension throughout your arms and shoulders. Also this exercise creates flexibility in the muscles of your shoulders, arms, and fingers.

INSTRUCTIONS

1. Choose one of the seated postures to begin. First, exhale all of the air stored in your lungs, and on your next inhalation, expand your chest as you stretch your

arms out to your sides and up over you head, with palms facing downward and outward as your arms are lifted up higher.

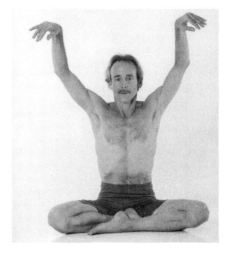

2. Move gracefully, with wrists slightly bent and soft, as if you were moving under water. After your lungs are completely full and your arms are up over your head, you will exhale and lower your hands and arms back down by your sides. Practice two or three repetitions, then relax and sit quietly for a few breaths.

The Pump—(All levels)

In this exercise you will look similar to an old-fashioned hand pump. This warm-up movement can also be used as a subtle *vinyasa* for select energy postures.

BENEFITS

This exercise releases tension and helps to create flexibility throughout your spine and neck. Also the pump will help to relieve gas and stomach cramps.

INSTRUCTIONS

1. Start by lying on your back in the Corpse Posture with your arms and legs extended out onto the floor.

2. On an inhalation, stretch your body long in both directions, lifting your arms up over your head.

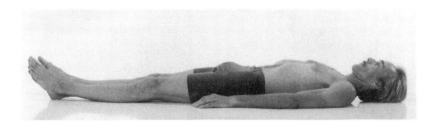

3. On an exhalation, tuck your left knee into your chest, as you hug your knee with your arms. Strive to touch your nose to your knee. Now inhale, release your grip, and stretch your body long once again. Repeat the same exercise on the opposite side to complete one round. Repeat the process, and then relax on your back for a few breaths.

Standing Body Twisting—(All levels)

This is a spinal and body twist practiced from a standing position. This exercise is a close relative to the Willow Tree which follows.

BENEFITS

This exercise relieves tension along your spine and throughout your torso. It also creates heat and flexibility needed to assist you in other yoga postures.

INSTRUCTIONS

1. Stand with your feet a little more than shoulder-width apart. Twist and rotate your torso from right to left in a slow, yet steady pace, allowing your arms to swing free as you move your body from right to left.

2. Practice two to four repetitions. When finished stand quietly and relax for a few breaths with your arms relaxed by your sides.

Standing Forward Bend (Uttanasana)—(All levels)

In Sanskrit *uttana* relates to an intense stretch. In this warm-up posture you will stand upright, reaching for the sky, then bend forward at the waist for a great warm-up stretch.

BENEFITS

In the Standing Forward Bend you will be creating length between the vertebrae. In addition you are stretching all the muscles on the back side of your body, as you release stress and tension.

1. Start from Mountain Posture, where you stand with feet together, arms relaxed and extended down by your sides, with spine straight, showing good posture. Slightly pull your navel in to your spine and stand tall as if there were a beam of light lifting you upward from the top of your head. On an inhalation lift the energy upward as you raise your arms up over your head, stretching your body long.

2. Exhale, hinging forward at the waist as you move gently into your Standing Forward Bend. Allow the energy of gravity to help create length in your spine and strive to place your hands on the floor beside your feet, with legs straight, yet not hyper-extended or locked.

3. **Beginners** can bend your knees slightly and rest your hands on your thighs, or shins. Hold this posture for five complete breaths. When finished, inhale and return to standing in Mountain Posture.

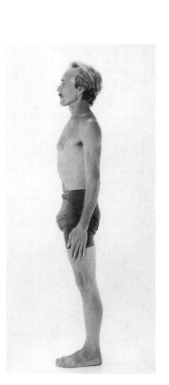
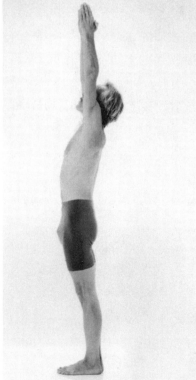
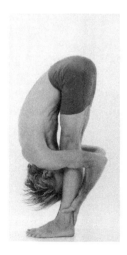

Willow Tree (Vrksasana-III)—(All levels)

This is a spinal and body twist practiced from a standing position. In this exercise you will resemble a willow tree swaying in the breeze.

BENEFITS

This exercise relieves tension along your spine and throughout your torso. It also creates some basic heat and flexibility needed to assist you in your yoga *asanas.*

INSTRUCTIONS

1.   Stand with your feet a little more than shoulder-width apart, letting your arms hang free as you bend your torso from right to left in a slow, yet steady pace. Allow your arms to swing free, with neck relaxed as you sway your body from right to left. Exhale as you bend your torso, inhale as you straighten your torso.

2.   On an inhalation lift your arms up over your head. Now exhale as you stretch your arms and torso to the left, slowly lifting your arms back up over your head on a inhalation, then exhale and stretch your arms and torso to your right side, When finished, stand quietly and relax for a few breaths.

Rocking the Baby (Preparation for Lotus)—(All levels)

Doing this exercise, you look like a parent gently rocking a baby from side to side to soothe and quiet the baby's spirit.

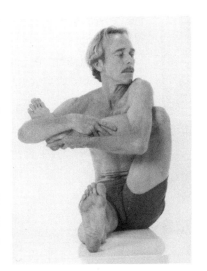

BENEFITS

Rocking the Baby will open your hips and create more flexibility in your knees and ankles.

INSTRUCTIONS

1.   Start from Seated Angle, bend your left knee, and cradle your leg with your arms, pulling it into your chest like you are holding a baby. Hold this posture and start your slow deep breathing.

2. Rock your bent leg from right to left with a gentle smooth motion as you continue your slow deep breathing. Practice three or four repetitions.

3. On an exhalation pull your left bent leg in toward your chest, up as high toward your shoulders as possible, releasing tension on exhalations, and hold for a few breaths. When finished, lower your leg back to the floor and repeat same steps with the right leg.

Cat Stretch—(All levels)

When practicing this warm-up exercise, you will resemble a cat stretching after a nice long nap. This warm-up movement can also be used as a subtle *vinyasa* for select energy postures.

BENEFITS

The Cat Stretch tones, strengthens, and stretches your back muscles and can make your entire spine feel stronger and more flexible. If you suffer from minor back pain brought on by stress, overactivity, or bad posture, this exercise can greatly help relieve that pain.

INSTRUCTIONS

1. Start by resting on your hands and knees. If you have sensitive knees, place an extra pad underneath each knee for support. Keep your toes pointed, your back should be straight (like a tabletop), but not rigid, and you should be supporting your weight equally between your hands and knees. Relax as you take three slow, deep breaths.

2. On an exhalation, arch your back up like a cat. Relax your neck as you drop your head downward and gaze toward your knees.

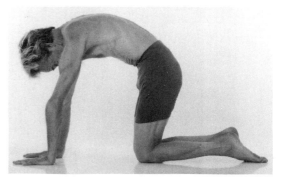

3. On an inhalation, sway your back, expanding your chest toward the ground, as you press your chest downward. Bend your arms to lower

your chest and bring your chin to rest on the floor between your hands.

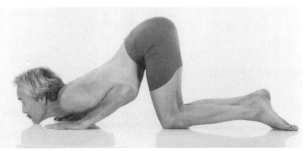

4. Exhale, and slowly return to the arched position you entered in Step #2.

5. On an inhalation, sway your back and expand your chest once again, only this time keep your arms straight and lift your head upward, as you extend your left leg backward and upward and your right arm forward. Don't swing or jerk into this posture: try to keep your movements fluid and soft as you move with the energy of your breath, lifting your head and extending your leg back and up at the same time.

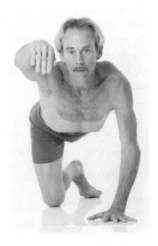

6. On an exhalation, lower your right hand to the floor, at the same time tucking your left knee into your chest, striving to touch your nose to your left knee.

7. On an inhalation, lower your left knee to the floor and once again sway your back, bending your elbows and allowing your chin and chest to touch the floor, then exhale and arch your back once again.

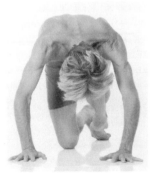

8. Now repeat Steps 5–7, only this time extending your right leg back and left arm up. **Beginners** should practice one or two repetitions with each leg, while **intermediate and advanced** can practice three or four rounds.

9. When finished, relax your torso onto your thighs, resting your hips on your heels, while extending your arms on the floor above your head, and rest your forehead on the floor in Child's Posture.

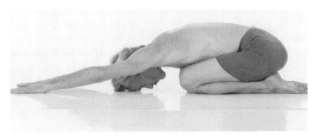

Sun Salutations (Suryanamaskar)—

The Sun Salutation is actually a combination of several different yoga postures connected together with a *vinyasa*, and serves as one of the best-known yoga warm-up exercises.

The Sanskrit word for Sun Salutation is *Suryanamaskar*. *Surya* means "sun" and *Namaskar* means "blessing, prayer or salutation." The Sun Salutation is an important Yoga exercise and is a healthy way to pay respect to the sun and at the same time salute the ultimate good within each of us.

TYPES OF SUN SALUTATIONS

Though all Sun Salutations share the same purpose and benefits, there are various forms of the exercise that require different levels of energy. There are soft-form and hard-form Sun Salutations. The hard-form Sun Salutations take a little more energy than the soft-form versions, and create more heat and build greater strength.

Level #1 (Beginner-Intermediate) Soothing Touch Salutation—

The Soothing Touch Salutation is perfect for beginners and takes a minimal amount of energy. Regardless of your level of practice, you will find this basic Sun Salutation very tranquil, fun, and beneficial.

This is basically a close relative to the traditional Sun Salutation, and is used in many soft-form styles of yoga practice. I have added a few subtle movements in order to enhance the energy flow and create a more soothing touch. This Sun Salutation is also the base for the other more elaborate Sun Salutations which follow.

BENEFITS

The Soothing Touch Sun Salutation benefits your whole body. The stretching and counter-stretching of the torso rejuvenates your spine to help relieve back pain. The Sun Salutation stretches and strengthens your arm and leg muscles and promotes flexibility in your ankles, knees, and hip joints. The gentle, fluid transition from stretch to counter-stretch combined with yoga breathing techniques leaves your mind in a very tranquil, yet alert and focused state. The Sun Salutation also rewards you with enhanced energy flow throughout your whole body and mind. As you practice your Sun Salutation remember to try and create a continuous movement from one posture to the next, like a slow dance.

INSTRUCTIONS

1. Start this posture by standing straight, relaxed, and firmly grounded with your feet together, spine straight, and shoulders back. Draw your navel in toward your spine and allow your arms to hang relaxed down by your sides. Direct your point of gaze forward and stand strong in Mountain Posture.

2. Take a few slow, deep breaths to calm and relax your mind. On an inhalation lift your arms up slowly in front of your body, with your wrists soft, as you move with fluid motion in a strong yet relaxed pace, as if you were moving under water. Time your movement so that fully raising the arms takes the same amount of time as your inhalation as you lift your arms up over your head. Arch slightly backward, and direct your gaze toward your hands. This is called Expanded Mountain Posture.

3. On an exhalation, slowly change directions as you move toward your Standing Forward Bend. Now your wrists are bent backward, arms extended and moving forward in a slightly circular movement. Continue your exhalation as you move further into your maximum Standing Forward Bend. If you find this stretch too intense, and have trouble keeping your knees straight, or are feeling tension in your back, try keeping your knees slightly bent and raise your hands to your shins or thighs.

4. On an inhalation, take a very large step backward with your right leg, as you inhale and let your right knee rest on the floor. Place both your hands on either side of your left foot. Arch your torso upward as you gaze toward the sky. Your hands are still on the floor on either side of your left foot. Your left leg is bent at 90 degrees or more, and your right leg is extended behind you, with your foot flexed, toes turned downward.

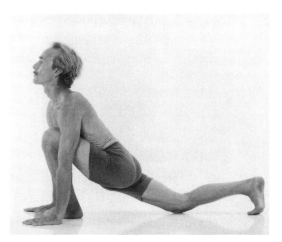

5. **Beginners** skip this move and go on to Step 6. **Intermediate to advanced** students can continue your inhalation as you expand your chest and lift your arms in a transition backward and upward in a circular motion, ending with palms together, and your head tilted with your vision up toward your hands. Exhale and lower your hands in prayer fashion, then return your hands to the floor.

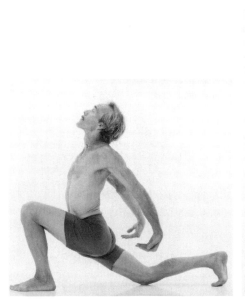

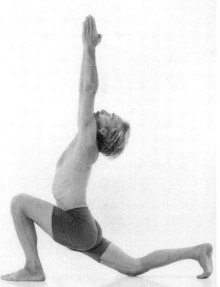

6. Exhale as you step back with your left leg to place it beside your right leg behind you, into Plank Posture. Move through the Plank Posture, let your knees stay slightly bent and resting on the floor, as you exhale all your air and lower your chest to the floor. Your arms should be stretched out on the floor in front of you and your hips over your calf muscles, with your torso resting on your thighs, as you move into the Child's Posture.

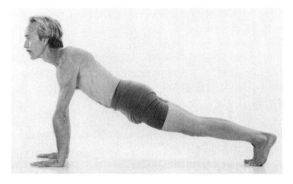

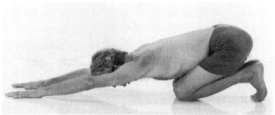

7. Start your inhalation and lower your torso onto the floor, passing out of the Child's Posture. Your hands are up under your shoulders, your knees slightly bent, your chest is resting on the floor, and your feet are pointed and resting on tops of your feet, into the Caterpillar Posture.

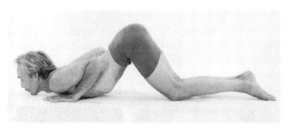

8. On an inhalation, pull your torso forward with your arms, as you push with your feet. Arch your body upward, moving into the Cobra Posture.

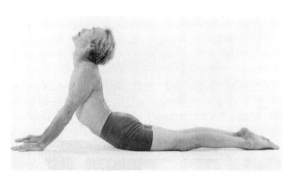

9. On an exhalation, retrace your steps as you lower your torso back down to the floor and pass through the Caterpillar Posture. Continue the exhalation as your lift your hips up into the air, pushing your body up by straightening your legs and arms. Your body will form a 90-degree angle from hips to hands and hips to feet as you move into the Downward Facing Dog Posture.

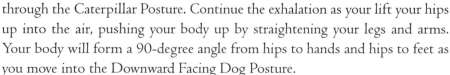

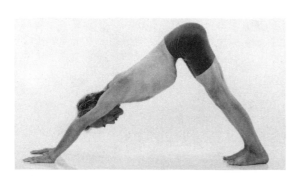

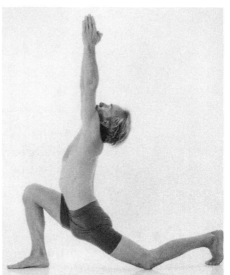

10. On an inhalation, step your right leg forward, up between your hands. Arch the torso upward, as you gaze toward the sky, opening the chest. **Beginners** go on to the next step; **intermediate to advanced** students can continue your inhalation as you expand your chest and lift your arms outward and upward over our head in a circular motion, ending with palms together, and your head tilted upward with your vision up toward your hands.

11. As you exhale step your left foot forward, moving back into the Standing Forward Bend.

12. On an inhalation, shift your body slightly forward in a wave-like motion to return to a standing posture. At the same time lift your arms up in front of your body, keeping your wrists soft and relaxed, with your hands extended over your head, arching your back softly.

13. Lower your arms down over your chest, in prayer fashion, as you exhale and stand straight as you return to the Mountain Posture.

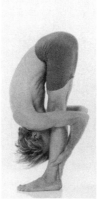

Repeat this same exercise twice. The second time begin by stepping back with your left leg first in Step 4.

Level #2: (Intermediate to Advanced) Ultimate Power Salutation—

If you want a great workout with your salutation, you can take on the Ultimate Power Salutation. This salutation takes full power and generates enough heat and energy to melt the snow off your driveway. The Ultimate Power Sun Salutation is very beautiful and can greatly help you to develop maximum strength and stamina. For those who want to sample this salutation, I have listed some modifications within the following instructions.

INSTRUCTIONS

I. Start Mountain Posture, with hands in prayer fashion over your chest. As you inhale, bend your knees, and in one fluid motion lower your hands down in front and then to the sides of your torso and slightly behind you. You should resemble a ski racer, slightly bent forward at the waist, expanding your chest with your gaze toward the Earth. Continue lifting your arms outward and upward all the way over your head, bringing your palms together and gazing at your thumbs. At the same time, bend your knees as if you were sitting in an imaginary chair.

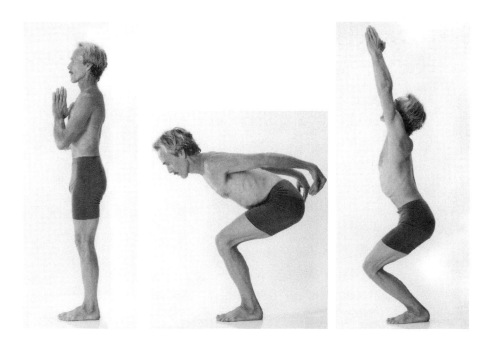

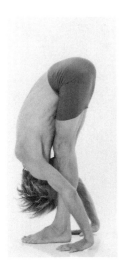
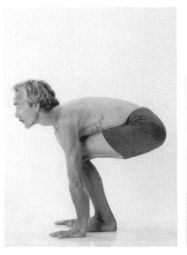
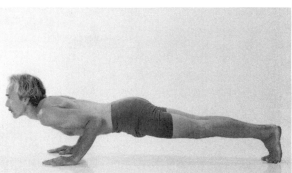

2. On an exhalation, bend forward and keep your chest open, leading with your heart as you move into a Standing Forward Bend.

3. On an inhalation, keep your hands on the floor as you arch your back and expand your chest. Direct your gaze upward. Bend your knees and prepare to step, or jump both legs back, landing with your body firmly in the Four Limbed Staff. **Beginners**, or those with other physical restrictions, may step back one foot at a time, instead of jumping. Exhale and lower your whole body to the floor moving into the Four Limb Staff.

4. On an inhalation, pull your torso forward with your arms and push with your feet. You will be arching your body upward into the Upward Facing Dog Posture. Push forward, rolling up onto the tops of your feet, lifting your torso upward, expanding your chest and opening your shoulders as you gaze upward.

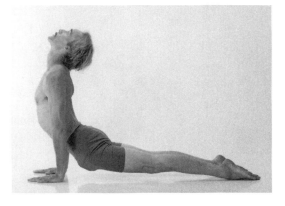

5. On an exhalation, lift your hips up into the air, as you drop your head and shoulders down, moving into the Downward Facing Dog Posture. Spread your

fingers wide, roll your shoulders outward and lift your hips into the air. Your arms and legs should be fully extended, your chest open, and your gaze directed toward your toes. Keep your feet about 12 inches apart and try to lower your heels to the floor. If you have trou-

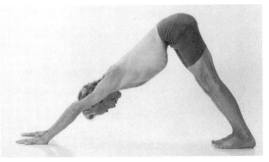

ble lowering your heels to the floor, walk your feet in toward your hands and bend your knees slightly. Those who want a lighter workout skip Steps 6–13 and resume with Step 14.

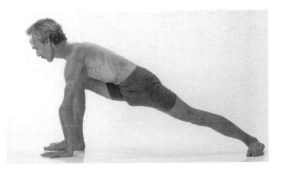

6. On an inhalation, turn your left foot sideways by pivoting on the ball of your foot and bringing your heel in toward the right foot. Take a large step forward with your right foot, placing your right foot on the floor between your hands. Try to position your knee over your ankle and your thigh parallel to the floor. Expand your chest, as you lift your torso up off your thighs. Lift your arms out to your sides and up over your head. Touch your palms together and gaze upward as you move into the Full Warrior I posture. In the transition from Downward Facing Dog to Warrior I Posture, strive to move on one inhalation. However, while you are learning this posture you should go ahead and take extra breaths if it is necessary.

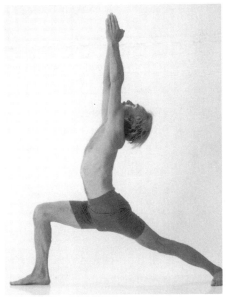

7. On an exhalation, lower your arms down to your sides, resting on either side of your right foot, then lower your body back to the floor, as you step your right leg back behind you, and lower your whole body into the Four Limb Staff.

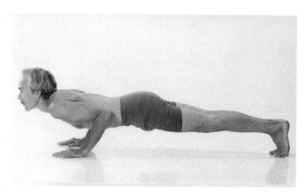

8. On an inhalation, pull your torso forward and arch your body up into the Upward Facing Dog Posture. Push forward, rolling up onto the tops of your feet, lifting the torso upward, expanding your chest and shoulders as you gaze forward.

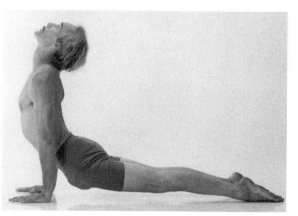

9. On an exhalation, lift your hips up into the air as you drop the head and shoulders down on an exhalation, moving into the Downward Facing Dog Posture. Spread your fingers wide, roll your shoulders outward and lift your hips into the air. Your arms and legs should be fully extended, your chest open, and your gaze directed toward your toes.

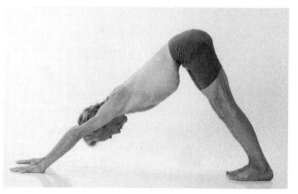

Keep your feet about 12 inches apart and try to lower your heels to the floor.

10. On an inhalation, turn your right foot sideways, pivoting on the ball of your right foot and bringing your heel in toward the left foot. Take a large step for-

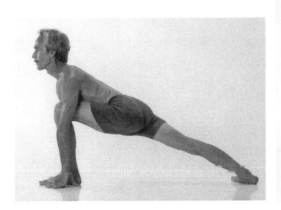
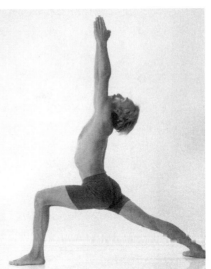

ward with your left foot, ideally placing your left foot up between your hands. Try to place your knee over your ankle, with your thigh parallel to the floor. Expand your chest as you lift your arms out to your sides and up over your head, fully extended in the Warrior I Posture. Again, try to move into this posture from Downward Facing Dog, all on one inhalation, but take more breaths if necessary.

11. On an exhalation, lower the extended arms down to your sides, placing your hands on the floor on either side of your left foot, as you step your left leg back behind you, lengthening the whole body into the Plank Posture; continue the exhalation as you lower your body down into the Four Limb Staff.

12. On an inhalation, pull your torso forward once again, pushing with your feet, rolling up on top of your feet and into the Upward Facing Dog Posture. You will be lifting your hips and dropping your head and shoulders back.

13. On an exhalation, lift your hips up into the air, as you drop the head and shoulders down, moving into the Downward Facing Dog Posture. Spread your fingers wide, roll your shoulders outward, and lift your hips into the air. Your arms and legs should be fully extended, your chest open, and your gaze

directed toward your toes. Keep your feet about 12 inches apart and try to lower your heels to the floor. Hold this position for five complete breaths. If you have weak wrists, elevate the palm of your hands one or two inches up off the floor with a rolled towel or a small wedge incline.

14. On an inhalation, jump (or step for a lighter workout) your feet back up between your hands, and exhale when you land. Bend forward into the Standing Forward Bend.

15. On an inhalation, lift your torso upward, pulling your arms out to your sides and up over your head, as you expand your chest, bending your knees as if you were going to sit down into a chair. Exhale and return to standing, lowering your arms down by your sides, as you straighten your legs, coming back to the Mountain Posture.

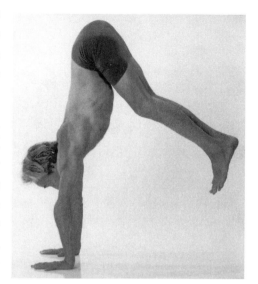

CATEGORY #3:
INVERTED POSTURES AND COUNTER STRETCHES

Headstand (Sirsasana)—(Intermediate to Advanced)

Sirsa means "head." In this posture you will balance on your head, supported by your arms. The Headstand is considered to be one of the main postures, due to its wonderful calming and relaxing effect on your whole body. The Headstand is an intermediate to advanced posture; however, anyone can practice the preliminary variations.

Caution: Inverted postures should be avoided if you have any of the following physical conditions:

- *a floating retina*
- *during your menstrual cycle*
- *severe injury to your neck*
- *glaucoma*
- *extreme high blood pressure*

BENEFITS

The Headstand posture helps you develop balance, self-confidence, and forearm strength. All of the inverted postures work on your body's cardiovascular system. When you place your body in an upside-down posture, you ease the flow of blood to your heart and brain. Combined with yoga deep breathing (which increases the oxygen supply to your blood), this concentration of fresh, oxygenated blood pulsing through your heart and brain leaves you feeling refreshed, at peace, yet very powerful.

INSTRUCTIONS: TRANSITION FLOW

1. Start your Headstand from the Folded Leaf Posture, with your knees bent, sitting with hips on your heels and your torso on your thighs. Your arms should be extended on the floor beside your torso, with palms facing upward.

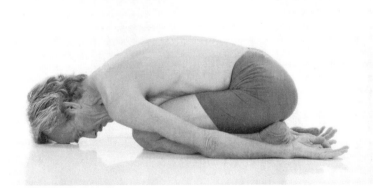

2. On an inhalation, start lifting your torso off your thighs, expanding your chest, as you begin to lift the energy upward, allowing your buttocks to raise up off

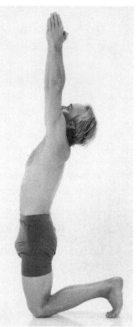

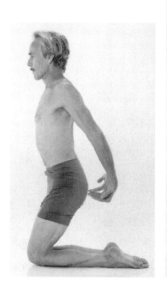

your heels as you lift your arms up over your head, with palms touching together, with your vision upward.

3. Start your exhalation as you lower the energy down toward the Earth, with your hands in prayer fashion. Bend your elbows, lowering your body down onto your forearms, interlacing your fingers, but leaving your hands cupped.

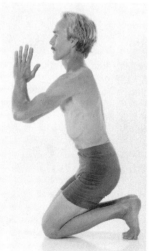

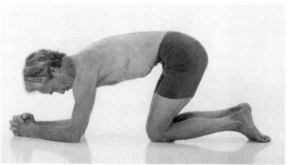

4. Lower your head onto the floor until you can place your cupped hands around the back of your head.

5. Support most of your weight on your elbows, making sure to keep your elbows close to parallel. Straighten your legs slowly, as you distribute your weight evenly between your supporting elbows and your feet. If you're not ready for a full Headstand, follow Steps 1–5, then relax into Child's Posture.

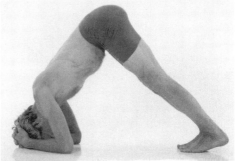

6. Slowly continue walking your feet up higher until your torso is almost vertical to the floor. If you are not absolutely confident about your balance, try the Headstand with your back against a wall for added support.

7. Bend your left knee, tucking it into your chest as you lift your left foot up off the floor. Then bend your right knee into your chest as you pull your right foot up off the floor. You can now straighten your legs up into a full Headstand. Hold this pose from five to twenty breaths, or longer if you are comfortable. Enhance your Head-stand by tucking your hips under, flattening your back and trying to form a straight line from your

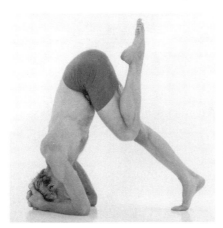

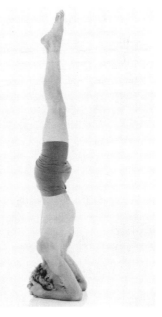

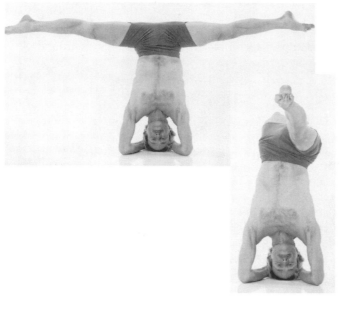

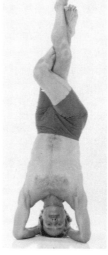

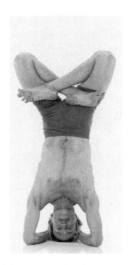

head through your spine and on through your toes. Avoid arching your back and pushing your stomach out: this could strain your back muscles.

8. **Advanced** students try the following more challenging variations: splitting your legs side to side, splitting your legs front to back, inverted Eagle Posture, full lotus twist.

9. When finished come down slowly: on an exhalation bend your knees into your chest and lower your torso back down onto your thighs, into Child's Posture.

Shoulder Stand (Salamba Sarvangasana)—(All levels)

Salamba means "propped or supported," *sarva* means "whole or complete," and *anga* means "limb or body." In this posture you will support your body with your hands and elbows.

This posture has acquired the appropriate name of Shoulder Stand, as you will balance your body on your shoulders.

BENEFITS

The Shoulder Stand stimulates the endocrine system and the thyroid and parathyroid glands are given a tune-up. When upside down you will receive an easy blood supply to your heart and brain and help to reverse the effects of varicose veins. When you come out of the Shoulder Stand, you will feel refreshed and rejuvenated.

TIPS AND CAUTIONS

1. If you are a beginner or have a sensitive neck, place a blanket under your shoulders to create a few inches of additional elevation. This will help protect your neck from injury. If you find it difficult to support yourself in a Shoulder Stand, another alternative is to start your Shoulder Stand with your legs running up a wall. In this manner you can bend your knees and push against the wall with your feet to give you added support.

INSTRUCTIONS: POSTURE FLOW

2. On an inhalation, stretch your body long in both directions, then exhale, bending your knees, lifting your feet up off the floor, as you move your knees up over your chest. Inhale as you lift your hips up off the floor, supporting with your hands up under your hips. Straighten your legs toward the ceiling.

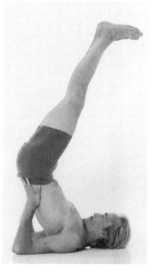

3. **Beginners** can start by lying down on your back with your legs extended up a wall, then bend your knees push-

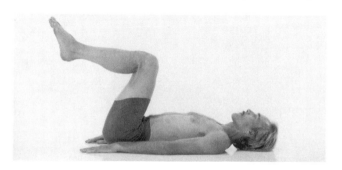

ing against the wall with your feet, as you use the wall for support to hold you in your Shoulder Stand.

5. Tuck your elbows behind your back so that they are parallel to one another, lifting your feet up toward the ceiling, and tucking your chin down into your chest. More advanced students can try to extend their legs and torso up as vertically as possible, placing your hands up behind your back to support yourself. Hold this posture from five to twenty very slow deep breaths.

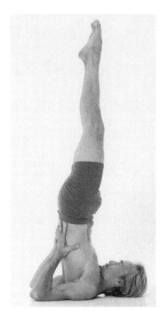

6. **Beginner to Intermediate:** When you are finished, place your hands back on the ground behind your back. Exhale and come down slowly, bending your knees and lowering your feet flat onto the floor. Then straighten your legs, lie back into the Corpse Posture, and relax.

Shoulder Stand Variations

INSTRUCTIONS

7. From the Shoulder Stand, lower your left leg down toward your head, keeping your foot flexed and leg straight, your right leg pointing straight upward. Strive to keep your hips squared and your torso vertical. Hold this posture for two or three complete breaths, then trade legs for another three complete breaths.

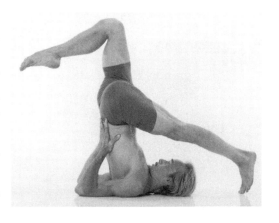

8. From the Shoulder Stand, bend your knees and place your feet on alternate thighs, for full Lotus Posture, then place hands on knees and balance.

9. When you are finished, place your hands back on the ground behind your back. Exhale and come down slowly, bending your knees and lowering your feet flat onto the floor. Straighten your legs, then lie back into the Corpse Posture and relax.

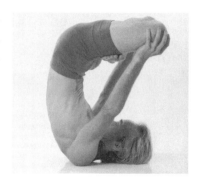

Plough Posture (Halasana)—

(Intermediate)

In the Sanskrit language the word *hala* relates to a plough, and in this posture your body will take on the appearance of a farmer's plough.

BENEFITS

The Plough Posture creates a toning and stretching effect along the entire back side of your body from the back of your neck to your feet. This posture will create a calm and relaxed state of mind, as it also restores energy.

INSTRUCTIONS

1. From the Shoulder Stand, exhale as you lower both legs down toward your head, and allow your arms to extend straight on the floor behind you with palms facing downward in Plough Posture. Hold this pose for five complete breaths. Allow your body to be in a neutral state as the energy passes through you.

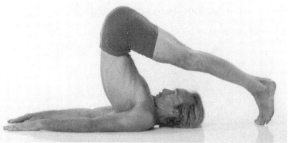

2. When you are finished, place your hands back on the ground behind your back. Exhale and come down slowly, bending your knees and lowering your back down gently onto the floor. Straighten your legs, then lie back into the Corpse Posture and relax.

Bridge Posture (Setu Bandhasana)—(All levels)

Setu means "bridge." In this posture you will resemble an arching bridge with supports. This posture is also used as a wonderful counter-stretch for the Headstand.

BENEFITS

In the Bridge Posture you will stretch and release tension from your chest, shoulders, arms, and thighs. This posture is an excellent counter-stretch for the Shoulder Stand and can be used as an alternative for the Fish Posture for those who have neck problems.

INSTRUCTIONS: TRANSITION FLOW

1. Lying down in the Corpse Posture, inhale, gathering energy, as you stretch lift your arms out to your sides and up over your head. Now exhale, lowering your arms back to your sides, bending your knees and placing your feet flat onto the ground with your hands by your sides, palms facing downward.

POSTURE FLOW

2. On an inhalation, lift your hips up toward the sky. Place your hands underneath your back on the floor below your hips. **Advanced** students can move into the Bridge Posture directly from the Shoulder Stand by exhaling and allowing your legs to gently flow to the floor behind your back.

3. Try to interlock your fingers as they push your hands down into the floor and lift your hips up toward the ceiling, stretching out your thighs and expanding your chest. **Advanced** students can hold your ankles. Hold this posture, doing your slow deep breathing for five breaths. When finished, lower your hips to the floor on an exhalation, as you unclasp your hands, relax, and return to Corpse Posture.

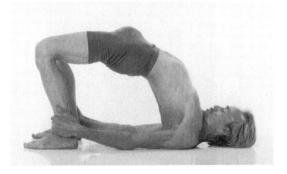

4. If you are a **more advanced** student, you can inhale and stretch your body long from Corpse Posture, then exhale returning to the Bridge Posture, only this

time try to lift your left leg up vertically toward the ceiling. You will be supporting your body weight with your left leg. Hold this posture for an additional two complete breaths, then relax, lower your body to the floor, and repeat on the opposite side. Flexible students can try to reach with both hands and grab the ankle of your supporting foot.

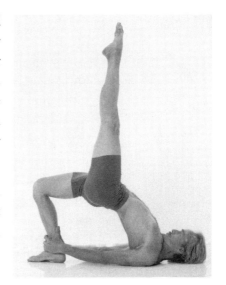

5. When finished on an exhalation, come down slowly and relax into Corpse Posture, laying flat on your back with your legs extended out in front of you.

Fish Posture (Matsyasana)—(All levels)

Matsya means a "fish." This posture is dedicated to the Hindu legend of *Matsya*, the fish incarnation of *Visnu*, who is the "source and maintainer of all things." This posture is also used as a wonderful counter-stretch for the Headstand.

BENEFITS

In the Fish Posture your thyroid gland is rejuvenated, due to the stretching of your neck. Your chest is expanded, and this helps greatly if you suffer from shallow breathing. This *asana* also serves to open the hips and release tension from your shoulders.

INSTRUCTIONS: TRANSITION FLOW

1. **Beginners** start from the Corpse Posture.

2. **Intermediate and advanced students** can remain lying down, and place their legs into Perfect Posture, or Lotus, with your hands by your sides. On an inhalation, gather the energy, as you lift your arms up over your head, stretching your body in both directions, then exhale and lower your hands down in prayer fashion over your chest.

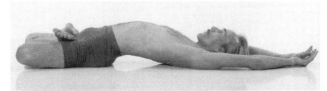

3. Arch your back up off the floor, expanding your chest, as you push down with your elbows, placing your hands on your thighs. **Beginners** should sit on top of your hands with your legs straight. Ideally try to lower the top of your head all the way to the floor.

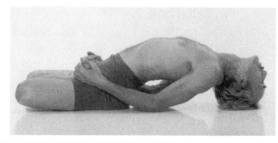

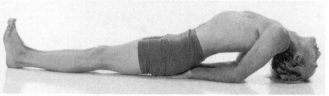

4. Stretch the whole front side of the body all the way up under your neck muscles. Hold this posture for five very slow deep breaths.

5. **Powerful Fish Variation** (Intermediate)—Remain in the Fish Posture and place your hands and arms extended about a foot up over your torso, with palms touching, as you lift your legs up off the floor on the same 45-degree plane.

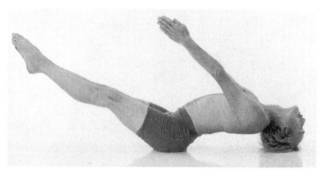

Hold for an additional five breaths: this is an excellent workout for your abdominal area.

6. When you finish an exhalation, take your hands out from underneath you, straighten your legs out, and lower your back to the ground, as you return to the Corpse Posture, lying flat on your back and relax.

Staff Posture (Dandasana)—(All levels)

Danda means "staff or rod." In this posture your arms on either side of your hips will resemble a staff or rod supporting your torso.

BENEFITS

In the Staff Posture, you will expand your chest, stretch the backside of your neck, enhancing posture and expanding lung capacity.

INSTRUCTIONS: TRANSITION FLOW

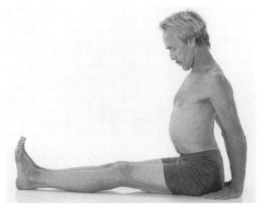

1. Start from the Seated Angle Posture, resting your hands on your extended legs. Inhale as you allow your hands to slide up your legs, drawing the energy upward, as you lift your arms up over your head, exhale and release the energy, parting the air up over your head, and lower your hands down into the floor by the side of your hips.

POSTURE FLOW

2. Begin with your palms facing downward beside your hips and your fingers pointing toward your toes. Drop your head forward like you were trying to look down at your navel; strive to place your chin all the way down into the notch in your chest. This chin pressure, into the notch in your breast bone, is the *Jalandhara bandha.*

3. Pull your shoulders backward and downward. Really expand your chest, exaggerating it, push your chest way out and arch your back. Flex your feet upward, close your eyes, and start doing your slow deep breathing for five deep breaths. *Staff Posture.*

4. When finished, inhale, lifting your arms up over your head, as in Step I, and look up at your hands. Exhale, lower your hands back down into your lap, and relax into Seated Angle Posture.

Seated Forward Bend (Paschimottanasana)—(All levels)

Paschima means "west." If your were standing facing the east, the whole front side of your body relates to the east and the whole back side of your body relates to the west. In this stretch you will stretch the whole back side of your body.

BENEFITS

In the Seated Forward Bend you will stretch and relax your muscles from the bottoms of your heels all the way up to the base of your skull. This posture stimulates nerves along your spine. The Seated Forward Bend is also used as a counter-stretch for back-bending postures.

INSTRUCTIONS: TRANSITION FLOW

I. You will start from the Seated Angle Posture, only resting hands in lap, sitting upright with your legs extended out in front of you. Exhale all of your air, and on your inhalation, expand your chest, lifting your arms out to your sides up over your head with palms facing away from each other.

2. After your lungs are completely full, you will exhale and lower your hands in prayer fashion, down over your heart. Now on an inhalation, interlace your fingers and stretch your arms up over your head.

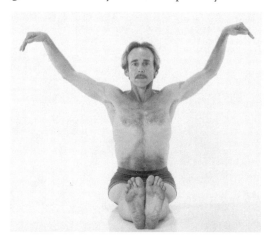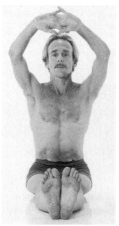

3. On an exhalation, start bending forward at your waist, circling your arms outward and downward toward your feet. Continue bending forward; if you cannot grasp on to your toes with your hands, just place your hands on top of your legs and bend your knees slightly to avoid rounding your lower back. You could also use a yoga strap or towel to extend your reach.

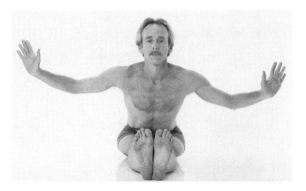

4. More flexible students, if it is possible, keep your back straight, leaning your torso out over your extended legs, folding flat onto your thighs. Grab on to your toes and hold for five very slow deep breaths.

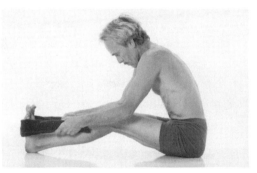

5. After you finish, inhale and start to sit back up into the Seated Angle Posture, letting your hands slide up your legs as you lift your torso upward. Lift your arms with soft wrists up over your head, as in Eagle Wings, com-

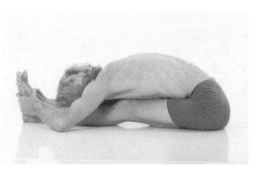

pletely filling your lungs with air. Exhale and lower your arms back down by your sides and relax into Seated Angle Posture with hands resting in your lap.

Incline Plane (Purvottanasana)—(Intermediate)

Purva means "east," relating to the whole front side of your body. In this posture you will stretch the body from under your chin to the tips of your toes.

BENEFITS

In the Incline Plane, you will stretch the whole front side of your body and strengthen your wrists, arms, and shoulders. This posture is used as the counter-stretch for the Seated Forward Bend.

INSTRUCTIONS: TRANSITION FLOW

1. Start from the Seated Angle Posture, with hands resting in your lap, sitting up straight on the floor with your legs extended fully out in front of you. Exhale all of your air, and then on the inhalation, expand your chest, lifting your arms out to the sides of your body and up over your head with palms facing outward, simulating an eagle as it stretches its wings. At the same time, keep your wrist soft and slightly bent, as if you were moving under water. Exhale as you lower your arms back down by the sides of your hips and slightly behind, as in Staff Posture.

POSTURE FLOW

2. **Beginners**—Bend your knees, with your feet flat on the floor, bringing your heels inward toward your buttocks, about a foot or so. Inhale, placing your hands on the ground, with fingers pointed toward your toes, your feet flat, lifting your hips up into the air, as you drop your head slightly backward. This is the beginning of the Incline Plane, which forms the shape of a tabletop.

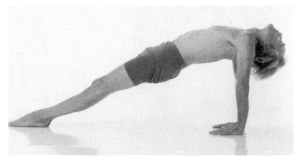

3. **Intermediate and advanced**— For those of you who are more advanced, try to keep your legs straight, extended fully all the way out, forming a 45-degree

angle from your feet on the floor to your raised head. Creating one straight incline plane with your whole body, from your toes all the way up to your forehead, like a giant ramp. Try to place your feet as close together as possible, with the soles of your feet flat on the ground and your head arched backward, as you stretch under the front of your neck. You should have your arms supporting your sides, fingers pointing toward your toes, as you lift your torso up off the ground. Ideally your torso will form a 45-degree angle with the ground, and your feet are flat on the floor.

4. Keep your hips up on that same plane, forming one long rigid incline plane with your whole body. Drop your head backward and continue with your slow deep breathing for five complete breaths.

5. When you finish, exhale, bending at the waist, lowering your hips back down to the floor, and return to the Seated Angle Posture with hands in lap. Exhale and relax.

Head Knee Posture I (Janu Sirsasana I)—(All levels)

Janu means "knee" and *sirsa* means "head." In this seated posture you will bend one knee, stretching forward and placing your head down over your extended knee.

BENEFITS

In the Head Knee Posture you stretch the muscles of your calf, hamstring, and shoulders, promoting mobility in your knee and hip joints. This posture also helps to relieve tension in your lower back, while enhancing proper function of your prostrate, spleen, and kidneys.

INSTRUCTIONS: TRANSITION FLOW

Beginners and intermediates can use this transition, **advanced** choose either Soft Touch *vinyasa*, or Muscle Power *vinyasa*, then return to Seated Angle when finished.

1. Start the Head Knee Posture preparation from Seated Angle Posture, sitting up straight with your legs stretched fully out in front of you, hands in lap.

2. Bend your left knee, placing your left foot against your right inner thigh, as you strive to place the heel of your left foot up near your perineum. Sit up straight with good posture and hands on right leg.

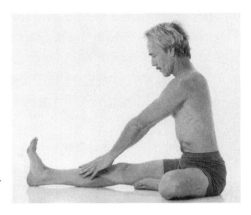

3. On an inhalation, lift the energy upward as you raise your arms upward, over your head, with your palms facing downward. At the same time soften your wrist, as if you were moving under water. On an exhalation, place your hands together in prayer fashion as you gather energy, lowering your hands down over your chest to your heart center. On an inhalation, interlace your fingers as you lift your arms up over your head, stretching your wrist and shoulders. Release your grip, hinge forward at your waist, as you circle your arms outward and forward, lowering your torso into a forward bend.

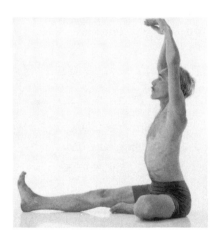
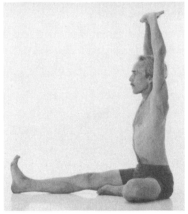
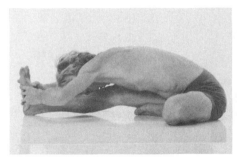

POSTURE FLOW

4. Try to lower your left knee down toward the floor, on your left side. **Beginners** might want to place a small pillow under your left knee. Your right leg is extended with your foot flexed.

5. Strive to reach the toes of your extended right foot, holding on to your foot with your fingers behind your foot and thumbs in front, pulling back on your extended right foot. **Beginners**: If this is not possible, you may use a strap to extend your reach.

6. Try to square your torso off in relationship to the extended left leg, lifting your right rib cage and lowering your left. If you are not very flexible, you may bend your right knee slightly or place a blanket up under your right knee.

7. Lift your elbows up, keeping your elbows slightly bent, drop your head down, and gaze down toward your right shin. Start doing your slow deep breathing for five complete breaths.

8. When you finish, on an inhalation, start lifting your torso, let your arms slide up your extended right leg, then lift your arms up over your head. Exhale and relax, moving the energy off to your sides, allowing your arms to return to your lap, as you straighten out your bent left leg and end in Seated Angle Posture. Now follow these same instructions on the opposite side, this time bending your right knee and bringing your right foot to left thigh.

Expanded Seated Angle (Upavistha Konasana)—*(All levels)*

The word *upavistha* means "seated posture," and the word *kona* refers to "an angle." In this variation of the Seated Angle you will have your legs stretched outward.

BENEFITS

In the Expanded Seated Angle you will stretch the muscles of your hamstrings, calves, and back. This posture also helps to circulate a healthy blood flow to your pelvic region and can often prevent a hernia.

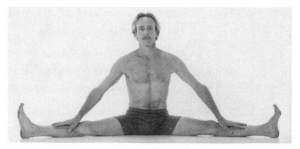

1. Start the Expanded Angle Posture from Seated Angle Posture, sitting up straight with your legs stretched fully out in front of you.

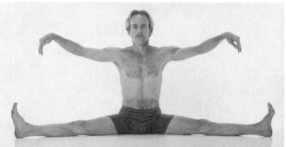

2. Now stretch both legs apart from one another until you have reached your maximum comfortable stretch.

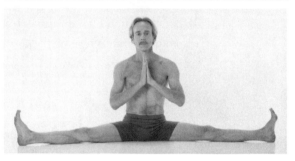

3. On an inhalation, lift your arms out to the side and upward, over your head, much like an eagle stretching its wings, with your palms facing downward. At the same time soften your wrists, as if you were moving under water. On an exhalation, place your hands together, in prayer fashion, as you lower your hands down over your chest to your heart center. On an inhalation, interlace your fingers, as you lift the energy, raising your arms up over your head, stretching your wrist and shoulders. Release your grip, hinge forward at your waist, as you try to lower your torso out over your right leg.

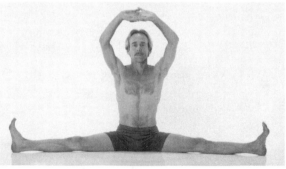

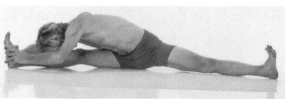

4. **Beginners** may keep your knees slightly bent, or place a pillow or blanket under your knees. Reach toward the toes of your extended right foot, with both hands. Hold your toes, with your thumbs in front and fingers behind, as you pull slightly backward. **Beginners** can use a strap to extend your reach.

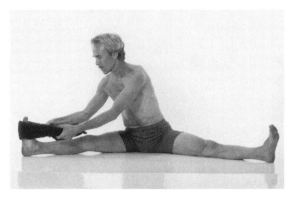

5. Hold this posture for five complete breaths and try to square your torso off in relationship to your extended right leg. When finished, inhale, lifting your arms up over your head, and raise your torso upright, exhale, and relax. Repeat the same exercise on the left leg. After you have stretched on each side, continue the next instructions to stretch forward.

6. Repeat the same transition flow as in Step 3, only this time you will stretch forward, striving to place your hands on the floor between your legs. If you are less flexible, place a pillow or bolster under your stomach for support.

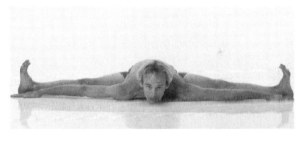

Advanced students may lay your torso flat on the floor and extend your arms parallel to your extended legs, with palms facing downward. Hold this position for five complete breaths, then inhale, lifting the energy upward, raising your torso and moving legs together, as you return to the Seated Angle Posture.

Flying Insect (Tittibhasana)—*(Advanced)*

Tittibha refers to a flying insect, and in this yoga posture you will take on the characteristics of a flying bug.

BENEFITS

This posture is a good leg stretch along with strengthening arms, shoulders, abdominals, and wrist. The Flying Insect also teaches balance, coordination, and the technique of "softness is strength."

INSTRUCTIONS: TRANSITION FLOW

Choose Soft Touch or Muscle Power *vinyasa* before you follow steps below.

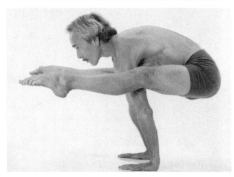

1. Begin in the Expanded Seated Angle Posture. When you are in the final posture, place your hands on the floor, under your knees. Bending your arms at the elbows, raise your legs. Feel the increase in the energy and relax and exhale. On an inhalation, lift your torso up into the Flying Insect Posture. For an extra stretch, lower your hips toward the ground and lift your feet upward.

2. Hold either of these postures for five complete breaths. When you are finished, exhale and lower your torso back to the floor and place your arms up on top of your extended legs. On an inhalation, let your arms slide up your extended legs, raise your torso, and continue lifting your arms up over your head; now exhale and relax. Allow your arms to return to

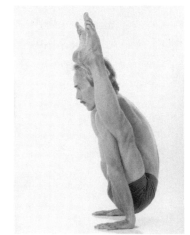

the floor as you move your legs and feet back together into Seated Angle Posture.

Shooting the Bow (Akarna Dhanurasana)— *(Beginner-Intermediate)*

In the Sanskrit language the preface *A* indicates the sense of closeness. The word *karna* means "ear," and *dhanur* refers to a bow. In this posture you will resemble an archer pulling the bowstring.

BENEFITS

In Shooting the Bow you will expand your chest and hips, stretch your hamstrings, and create mobility in your knee joints. This posture also strengthens your arms and relieves tension from your lower back.

INSTRUCTIONS: TRANSITION FLOW

I. Start the posture from the Seated Angle Posture, sitting up straight with your legs stretched fully out in front of you.

2. Place both hands on your extended legs. On an inhalation, allow your hands to slide up your legs, drawing the energy in toward your torso, as you lift your arms gracefully up over your head. On an exhalation, start to separate your arms up over your head, as you move the energy forward, bending your torso slightly forward, lowering your arms in a circular motion, downward and forward toward your extended toes. At the same time bend your left knee, placing your left foot up onto your right thigh. Grab the top of your left foot with 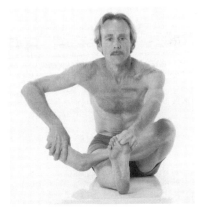 your right hand as you also grasp on to your right foot with your left hand.

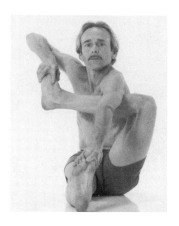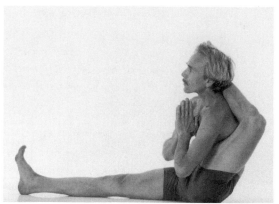

3. Strive to lift your left foot up toward your right ear, as you hold the toes of your right foot with your left hand. Hold this posture for five complete breaths. When finished, inhale as you release the grip on your toes, raise your torso, and lift your arms up over your head, then exhale and straighten your left leg, relax, and lower your hands back down to your legs into Seated Angle Posture. Repeat the same exercise on the opposite side. **Beginners** can use a strap to extend your reach on both feet.

4. **Advanced students only**: One Leg Behind Head—*Ek Pada Sirsasana*. Repeat Step 3, only this time you will place your leg behind your head, then place your hands in prayer fashion over your chest. Hold this position for three complete breaths. When finished, place your hands on the floor, pushing downward as you lift your hips off the ground and raise your extended leg upward. When finished, exhale and lower your hips and leg to the floor, then relax into Seated Angle Posture.

Boat Posture (Navasana)—(All levels)

The Sanskrit word *nava* translates as meaning "boat" or "ship," and in this posture you resemble a boat floating in the water. The Boat Posture is a good alternative for a full-power *vinyasa*.

In the Boat Posture you strengthen the muscles of your stomach, legs, and arms. This posture helps firm your waistline and tone your kidneys while you develop strength and power.

INSTRUCTIONS: TRANSITION FLOW

Beginners can use the Soft Touch *vinyasa*. **Intermediate to advanced** students can choose the same, or the Muscle Power *vinyasa*.

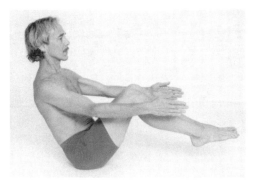

I. Start from the Seated Angle Posture, hands by your sides with legs extended out in front of your torso. Inhale, raising your arms up over your head using Eagle Wings. Exhale as you lower your arms, embracing the energy, bending your knees, and lift your feet up off the floor with your back straight, as you balance on your buttocks. Your arms are extended out parallel to the ground. Balance in this posture for three complete breaths.

POSTURE FLOW

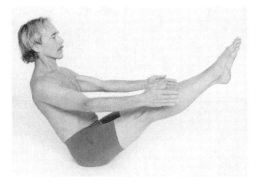

2. If you are comfortable with this posture, try straightening your legs, as you lift them to form a 45-degree angle with the floor. This leg-lift gives your stomach and legs an even greater workout. Hold this posture for five breaths and work up to three repetitions.

3. When finished, exhale, lower your legs to the floor, and relax into the Seated Angle Posture.

Cobra Posture (Bhujangasana)—(All levels)

Bhujanga means "snake or serpent." In this posture you will resemble a snake as it slowly uncoils, lifting its head and torso up into the air.

BENEFITS

The Cobra is a wonderful way to tone and strengthen the entire length of your spine, as it also helps to correct any vertebrae out of alignment, and can help correct bad posture.

INSTRUCTIONS: TRANSITION FLOW

1. Lie down on your stomach, arms by your sides, palms facing upward. Turn your head to the side and relax. Turn your head forward, resting your chin in to the floor, bend your elbows, placing your hands up under your shoulders; your feet are pointed, yet relaxed. **Beginners** try placing a pillow under your thighs for extra support.

2. On an inhalation, start slowly lifting the energy upward as you raise your shoulders and torso up off the floor, one vertebra at a time, resembling a snake slowly uncoiling. Lift up on an inhalation as high as is comfortable for your spinal flexibility. If you are not that flexible, you can rest on your bent elbows; if you are more flexible, lift your torso up higher by extending your arms fully; less flexible, keep your elbows slightly bent.

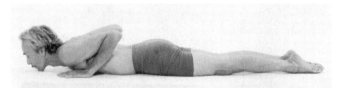

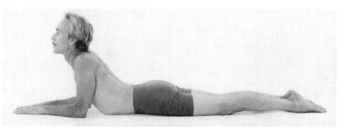

3. Keep your toes pointed and strive to leave your hips on the floor, feet together. When you reach your maximum comfortable stretch, then exhale and lower your torso back to the floor. Repeat this process three times, lifting up and stretching on an inhalation and lowering down on an exhalation. On your third round, hold your upward Cobra Posture for five deep breaths. If you have a stiff lower back you can separate your legs and feet a bit and allow your ankles to turn outward, or place a pillow up under your thighs.

4. Return your torso and shoulders back down to the floor, taking your hands out from under your shoulders, extending your arms back to your sides, and turn your head to the side and relax. Move into Child's Posture as a counter-stretch.

Upward Facing Dog (Urdhva Mukha Svanasana)—(Intermediate)

Urdva mukha means "upward facing" and *shvan* relates to a dog. In this posture you will resemble a dog stretching upward as it lengthens its legs and back after a nice nap. Upward Facing Dog is part of the Sun Salutation series.

BENEFITS

You will receive the same benefits as in the Cobra Posture, only with added strengthening for the muscles of your arms, back, abdominal, and shoulders. This posture is a good preparatory posture to strengthen you for the more strenuous *vinyasa* and serve as a base to enter and exit other yoga postures.

INSTRUCTIONS: TRANSITION FLOW

1. Follow the same instructions for Steps 1 and 2 as for the Cobra Posture, only this time you will engage muscles of your abdominal, back, and arms as you rest solely on the tops of your feet and your hands. Those with a stiff back may place a pillow under your upper thighs for support.

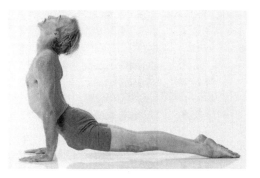

2. Hold this position for three to five complete breaths, then exhale and relax into the Child's Posture.

Half Locust (Ardha Salabhasana)—(All levels)

Ardha means "half" and *salabha* refers to the "locust" insect. In this posture you will feel the energy of the Earth as you rest on the ground, like a locust resting in the grass.

BENEFITS

This posture really helps to strengthen your lower back and can be very valuable in relieving back pain, as it also enhances proper alignment of your spinal disc. The Half Locust Posture helps to relieve flatulence.

INSTRUCTIONS: TRANSITION FLOW

1. Move through Cobra and Child's Posture before entering this posture. Inhale to enter Cobra, as you lift the energy upward, exhale, returning the energy to the Earth as you relax into Child's Posture, then inhale and lie down on your stomach.

POSTURE FLOW

2. Lie down on your stomach, with your arms extended by your sides, palms facing upward. Turn your head forward, resting your chin on the floor. You will stretch your chin in this posture, so if this causes discomfort, place a blanket under your chest to create an few inches of elevation, taking the pressure off your neck.

3. Place your arms down by your sides, with your hands placed up under your thighs, palms facing downward.

4. Stretch your chin out long, as though you are trying to look out in front of you. Exhale all your air first, and then, on inhalation, lift your left leg backward and upward, pressing down into the floor with your right foot. Hold this posture for five complete breaths, then practice the same exercise with your left

leg back and up. **Intermediate to advanced** follow the same instruction, only try extending your leg up higher and lifting your hips up off the floor, as you flex the supporting foot.

5.   Repeat two repetitions on each side, then exhale and relax onto your stomach.

Full Locust (Salabhasana)—(All levels)

You will lift both legs at the same time. Caution: This posture should not be attempted by anyone with a weak or injured neck.

BENEFITS

You will receive all the benefits of the Half Locust, with additional abdominal work, strengthening muscles of your lower and upper back along with stretching from the chest and neck.

INSTRUCTIONS: TRANSITION FLOW

1.   Start by lying down on your stomach, placing your arms down by your sides, with your hands placed up under your thighs, palms facing downward. On an inhalation, lift the energy upward as you move through Cobra Posture and then exhale into Child's Posture. Now inhale and return to the floor; exhale lying on your stomach.

POSTURE FLOW

2.   Unless you are experienced, try placing a folded blanket up under your chest and breastbone to reduce stress on your neck. Lie on your stomach with your arms extended underneath you, palms facing downward, resting your thighs on top of your hands; exhale all of your air. **Beginners and intermediate** can arch your torso, lifting your shoulders and knees up off the floor.

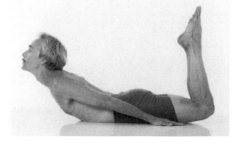

3.   **Advanced** students—This is a very difficult posture and should not be attempted by those who do not have some previous expe-

rience with yoga or have a very flexible back and strong stomach muscles. On inhalation, bend your knees, lifting both feet back up behind you, trying to thrust your whole torso up off the floor, lifting both feet up into the air, at the same time forming a vertical angle with the ground. Hold this posture for five slow complete breaths.

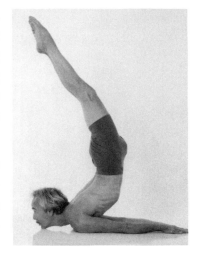

4. When finished allow your legs and torso to return to the floor. Relax, take your hands out from underneath you, turn your head to the side, and close your eyes and relax for a few seconds. As a counterstretch move into Child's Posture.

Bow (Dhanurasana)—(Intermediate)

Dhanu means a bow weapon. In this posture you will form an arched bow with your body, your arms acting as the bowstring as you hold on to your ankles.

BENEFITS

This posture helps to tone abdominal muscles and, with regular practice, assists in creating a very elastic spine. You will also open your shoulders as you stretch your thighs and expand your chest. This is a good posture to help overcome bad posture, and it can assist with correcting spinal alignment.

INSTRUCTIONS: TRANSITION FLOW

1. Start by lying down on your stomach, placing your arms down by your sides; turn your head to the side and relax. On an inhalation, lift the energy as you move through Upward Dog and exhale into Downward Dog, then inhale and return to the floor. Exhale, lying on your stomach.

POSTURE FLOW

2. Lie on your stomach with your arms extended by your sides and palms facing upward. Bend both of your knees, reaching back with your hands and trying to

grab your ankles with your hands. **Beginners** can use a strap to extend your reach.

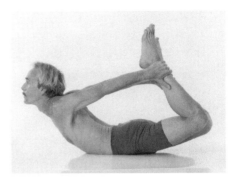

3. Hold this posture for five complete breaths, then relax back on to your stomach for a few breaths and repeat the exercise one more time. When you are finished, release your hands from your feet and return to your stomach, then take a counter-stretch, by resting into the Child's Posture for a few breaths.

4. **Advanced** students can try practicing the sideways bow by rolling your whole body over onto your right side for three complete breaths, looking over your right shoulder, up toward the ceiling. Then practice the same exercise on the opposite side for an additional three breaths. When finished relax into the Child's Posture.

Camel Posture (Ustrasana)—(All levels)

Ustra means "camel." In this backward-arching posture you will somewhat resemble a camel.

BENEFITS

The Camel helps to correct rounded shoulders and improves posture. It expands your chest and stretches the whole front side of your body, as you tone your whole spine

INSTRUCTIONS: TRANSITION FLOW

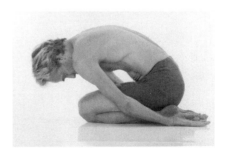

1. Begin in Child's Posture by sitting on your bent knees, with your torso resting on your thighs.

2. On an inhalation, embrace the energy, as you start lifting your torso upward from Child's Posture. Continue your inhalation until your arms are up over your head and your torso is upright and vertical to the floor.

3. On an exhalation, release the energy as you lower your arms down, placing your hands on your hips with your elbows bent. Gently arch your back, looking up toward the ceiling.

4. **Beginners** push forward on your hips and extend your torso backward, trying to look up toward the ceiling, creating length in your neck. Hold this posture for five complete breaths. When finished, inhale, lifting your torso upright, as you raise your arms up overhead; now exhale and relax back into the Child's Posture.

5. **Intermediate** students: Flex your feet and strive to place both hands down onto your heels. Hold this posture for five complete breaths. **Advanced** students, with feet pointed, place your palms against the soles of your feet. Hold this position for five complete breaths. When finished, inhale, lifting your torso upright, as you raise your arms up overhead. Now exhale and relax back into the Child's Posture.

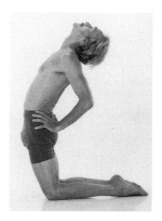 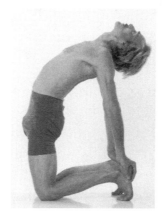 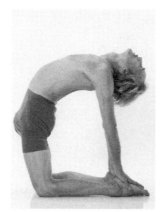

Upside Down Bow (Urdhva Dhanurasana)—(Advanced)

Urdhva means "upward" and *dhanu* relates to a bow. In this posture you will form an upside-down bow. This posture is often called the Wheel Posture, or Back Bend.

BENEFITS

This posture is excellent for creating a supple spine, expanding your chest, and strengthening your arms and wrists. It also helps to send oxygenated blood to your brain, leaving you with a very relaxed and refreshed feeling.

INSTRUCTIONS: TRANSITION FLOW

1. Choose either the Soothing Touch or Muscle Power *vinyasa* listed at the end of the chapter. After your *vinyasa*, enter the Corpse Posture, lying on the ground, extending your arms by your sides, palms facing upward; your feet should be about one foot apart.

POSTURE FLOW

2. Bend your knees and draw your feet up toward your hips, keeping your feet flat on the ground.

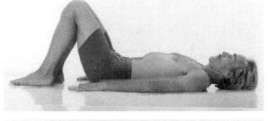

3. Raise your hands up by your ears and tuck your hands, palms down, under your shoulders. **Beginners:** Simply inhale, lifting your hips upward, arching your back up off the floor, as you leave your shoulders on the floor.

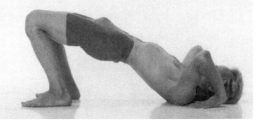

4. **Intermediate:** Exhale all of your air, then inhale, as you push down with your hands, trying to roll back up on top of your head. Take caution in this step, as it is very difficult if you have a weak neck. At the same time, lift your hips up into the air and arch your back. If you have weak or injured wrists, place a small two-inch lift under the palm of each hand. Align your

feet parallel with one another, distributing your weight evenly between both feet. Hold this posture for five to ten breaths, and try three repetitions.

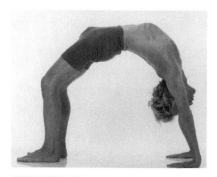

5. **Advanced** students continue pushing up with your hands and feet. Straighten your elbows and raise your hips until your body forms a large arch or wheel. For a challenging variation, lift your left leg up vertical to the floor, for three breaths on each side.

6. When finished, exhale and bend your elbows to lower your head down and then softly relax your whole body back down onto your back, in the Corpse Posture.

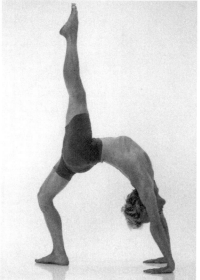

CATEGORY #6—TWISTING POSTURES

Spine Toner—(All levels)

The Spine Toner is easy to practice and a wonderful way to release tension in your back.

BENEFITS

The Spine Toner will invigorate your entire spine with a gentle twisting that stretches the muscles in your back and hips. Be sure to combine this exercise with yoga breathing techniques.

Starting from the Seated Angle Posture, inhale in Eagle Wings, then exhale lowering into Corpse Posture.

1. From Corpse Posture, extend your arms straight out from your shoulders, at a 90-degree angle from your torso. Become neutral as you absorb the energy from the Earth.

POSTURE FLOW

2. On an inhalation, lift your right leg upward toward the sky, then exhale, twisting your torso to the left and lower your right leg over your left leg toward the floor, on the left side of your body. If possible, keep your legs straight. If you find this posture uncomfortable, bend your right knee.

3. Strive to keep your shoulders flat on the floor as you turn your head and gaze to the right side of your torso.

4. Hold this posture for five complete breaths, then slowly inhale, lifting your right leg up toward the sky, then exhale and return it to its original position.

5. Repeat the same exercise on the opposite side. When finished, relax on your back in the Corpse Posture for five to ten slow, deep breaths.

Twist Posture I (Ardha Matsyendrasana)—(All levels)

In Hindu legend, Matsyendra was a fish which twisted around in order to hear the secrets of yoga from Lord Siva. Matsyendra was then incarnated in human form, in order to spread the knowledge of yoga. This posture is dedicated to Matsyendra, the twisted fish. In Sanskrit the word *ardha*, or "half," refers to the basic twist; the full twist is practiced in Lotus.

BENEFITS

Twist Posture I is a great way to tone and strengthen your spine. It can also assist in relieving backaches. It stretches the muscles in your shoulders, around your ribs, and in your neck, helping to relieve tension and leave you feeling invigorated.

Choose either the Soothing Touch or Muscle Power *vinyasa* from the floor to standing and back to the floor before starting this posture.

1. Start from the Seated Angle Posture, sitting on the floor with both legs extended out in front, your spine straight, and your shoulders back.

POSTURE FLOW

2. Bend your right knee and place your right foot over your left leg. Now bend your left leg in to bring your left foot up toward your right hip.

3. Lift your arms up and twist your whole torso to the right, moving in a graceful, flowing motion. Try to move your left elbow to the outside of your right knee. **Beginners,** place your right hand on the floor behind your back, with your left leg extended for support. In addition beginners will find this posture easier by placing a towel or small block under their left hip.

4. Strive to keep your torso upright and maintain breathing. Hold this posture for five complete breaths on each side.

5. **Intermediate to Advanced**—Reach your left arm under your right bent knee and strive to grab your left wrist behind your back. Repeat the same stretch and counter-stretch on the opposite side, then relax back into the Seated Angle Posture. Hold for five breaths on each side.

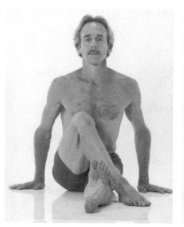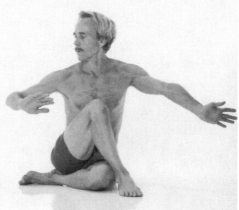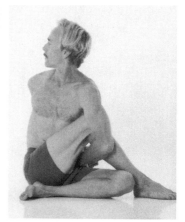

Noose Posture (Pashasana)—(Intermediate to Advanced)

The word *pasha* relates to a rope made into a noose. In this posture you will take on the appearance of a noose.

BENEFITS

In the Noose Posture you will stretch your Achilles tendons, tone and strengthen your spine, as well as removing tension from your lower back.

INSTRUCTIONS: TRANSITION FLOW

1. Starting from Mountain Posture, inhale and stretch your arms up over your head, embracing the energy, then exhale into a Standing Forward Bend.

2. Now inhale, bending your knees, and rest into a squatting position using your hands to support your hips.

POSTURE FLOW

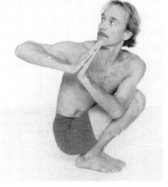

3. **Beginners and intermediate** students will find this posture easier by sitting on a yoga block. Twist your torso to your right side, placing your hands in prayer fashion, with your left elbow on the outside of your right knee.

4. **Advanced** students can wrap your left arm around both knees striving to grab your right wrist with your left hand. Hold this posture for five complete breaths on each side, then exhale as you move into Standing Forward Bend and inhale as you return to Mountain Posture.

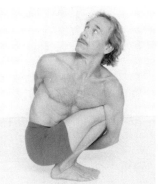

Plank Posture (High Push-up)—(Intermediate)

In this posture your body will form one very straight line, taking on the resemblance of a plank or board. The Plank and Four Limbed Staff postures form two links contained within the more powerful *vinyasa* and are good training.

BENEFITS

This is a preparation posture for the Four Limb Staff. It builds strength in arms and shoulders. It also assists in flattening the abdominal area and pectoral muscles. It serves as a nice muscle resistance exercise.

INSTRUCTIONS: TRANSITION FLOW

Begin with the Soft Touch *vinyasa*, ending in Thunderbolt Posture.

1.   Sit on the floor resting on your hands and knees, forming a tabletop with your back, as you exhale and arch your back like a cat.

2.   Now inhale and straighten your legs back behind you, one at a time, forming one line from your head to your toes, resting totally on your hands and feet with arms fully extended. Hold this posture for three to five complete breaths.

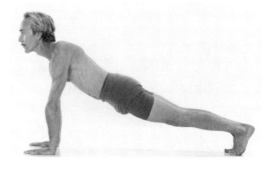

3.   **Four Limbed Staff:** Now bend your arms as you lower your torso and legs to a position about two inches off the floor. This is the Four Limbed Staff Posture. Hold this posture for an additional three to five complete breaths. When finished, relax into Child's Posture.

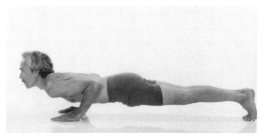

Downward Facing Dog (Adho Mukha Shvanasana)—(All levels)

Adho mukha translates as "facing downward" and *shvana* means "dog." In this posture the legs are strong and heels are lengthened, with your body resembling a dog stretching long after a nap.

BENEFITS

In Downward Facing Dog Posture, the heels and calves are stretched out and the muscles of legs, arms, and shoulders are strengthened. This is a great posture to help restore and maintain the body while reducing stiffness in the heels, ankles, and legs.

INSTRUCTIONS: TRANSITION FLOW

Use the Cat Stretch Posture as a *vinyasa* before practicing this posture.

POSTURE FLOW

1. Start by resting on your hands and knees, with your hips, back, neck, and head forming a straight line. Make sure your knees are directly under your hips and your hands are directly under your shoulders.

2. Come up on your toes and slowly begin straightening your legs to push your hips upward; as your legs straighten, drop your head down toward the ground. Keep your arms straight and elbows relaxed.

3. Try to lower your heels to the floor as your legs straighten; your feet should be about one foot apart. If you can't comfortably straighten your legs and your heels will not go to the floor, don't worry: leave your knees slightly bent and place a folded towel under the heels of your feet.

4. Without straining or locking your elbows or knees, you should try to create a nice 90-degree angle with your body as you make a straight line from your heels to your hips and another from your hips down your arms and to your hands.

5. Roll your shoulders outward, create some length in your spine, be strong yet relaxed. Gaze toward your toes and start taking very slow deep breaths; try to hold Downward Facing Dog for five to ten complete breaths.

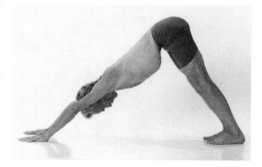

6. When finished, relax, lower your knees to the ground, fold your body in half, and relax into the Child's Posture.

Peacock Posture (Mayurasana)—(Advanced)

Mayur means "peacock." In this posture you will resemble the beautiful bird as it proudly struts across the meadow.

BENEFITS

This is a wonderful posture for strengthening your arms, shoulders, wrists, and your abdominal muscles.

INSTRUCTIONS: TRANSITION FLOW

1. Start in the Thunderbolt Posture, sitting upright, resting on your knees, with good posture. On an inhalation, lift your hips up off your heels, flexing your feet. At the same time lifting your arms outward and upward, similar to an eagle stretching its wings, as you lift your torso upward. On an exhalation, lower your hands down in front of your torso, with your hands in prayer fashion. Lower your palms down onto the floor, out in front and between your knees, with your fingers pointing toward your toes.

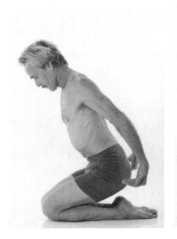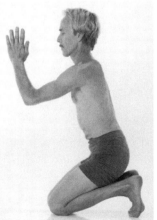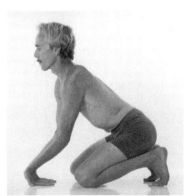

2. Bend your elbows back into and under your abdominal muscles, trying to place your elbows as close to your navel as you can. Turn your hands downward with your fingers facing back toward your knees. In order to take some of the tension off your wrist, push with your 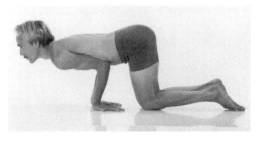 bent legs in a forward direction toward your head; this should assist in straightening your wrist a bit. Or you can also elevate the palms of your hands a few inches; this will also avoid any excessive pressure on your wrist.

3. Lift your head up, supporting yourself on your bent forearms with your elbows resting into your stomach muscles, straightening your legs all the way out. You are now resting on your toes and elbows, with your vision forward. 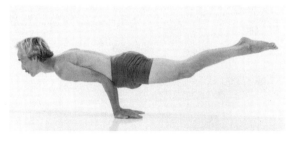 Ultimately, continue shifting your weight forward and try to lift your feet up off the floor, balancing your whole body parallel to the floor. If this is not possible, place your feet on a block.

4. Try to hold this position for five very slow deep breaths. If you find this too difficult on your wrists, you can turn your hands slightly outward with your fingers pointing out to the sides rather than pointing at your toes.

5. When you have finished, lower your legs to the ground, bending your knees, sit back into Child's Posture, and shake out your wrists in order to release any tension.

Scale Posture (Tolasana)—(Intermediate)

Tola means "pair of scales." In this *asana* you will resemble a scale as you balance your body's weight.

BENEFITS

Tolasana is an excellent posture for strengthening the muscles in your stomach, arms and shoulders. This posture is a great strengthening exercise and is sometimes used as a preparation for deep relaxation.

INSTRUCTIONS: TRANSITION FLOW

Start this *asana* from Perfect Posture. **Advanced** students can first move to standing and back to the floor through the *vinyasa* avenue of Soft Touch, or Muscle Power *vinyasa*.

POSTURE FLOW

1. **Beginners** sit on the floor in Perfect Posture. Advanced in full lotus posture. On an inhalation, lift your arms outward and upward all the way up over your head, then exhale and lower your arms to the floor.

2. Place your hands on the floor beside your hips. Now push down with your hands, lifting your torso off the floor. If you have difficulty, put some blocks under your hands to give you some extra lift.

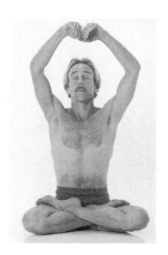
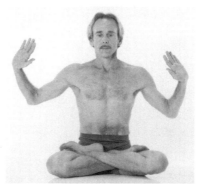
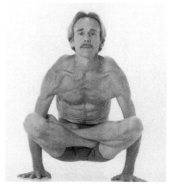

3. While your body is suspended, try lifting your knees up toward your chest; hold this position for five to ten complete breaths. **Advanced** students can take the legs out of Lotus and try another variation: with your legs straight, point them up toward the ceiling. This is the Flying V Posture.

4. When finished, lower your hips back to the floor, straighten out your legs, and relax into Corpse Posture.

Scorpion Posture (Vrishchikasana)—(Intermediate to Advanced)

The word *vrishchika* relates to a scorpion, and in this posture your body will resemble this insect. This posture is an intermediate to advanced posture and should not be attempted by beginners.

BENEFITS

In the Scorpion Posture you will strengthen your upper arms and shoulders while greatly enhancing your balance. The inverted nature of this posture will create a tranquil effect on your mind and teach you how softness is strength.

INSTRUCTIONS: TRANSITION FLOW

1. Start this posture from the Thunderbolt Posture, resting on your knees. Inhale, lifting your arms upward as in Eagle Wings as you embrace the energy, then exhale back to Thunderbolt Posture. Lean forward, placing your elbows and forearms flat on the floor in front of your knees.

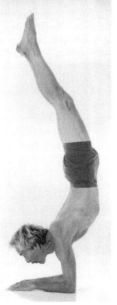

POSTURE FLOW

2. Lift your hips up off your knees as you straighten your legs, supporting half your body weight on your elbows and forearms and the other half on your feet. Now inhale and kick your feet upward to balance on

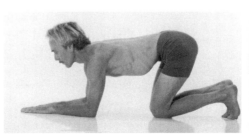

your forearms. Hold this posture for three complete breaths. **Advanced** students can press their legs up smoothly.

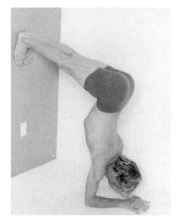

3. **Intermediate** students, or those who are practicing this posture for the first time, posture yourself with a wall behind your feet for support .

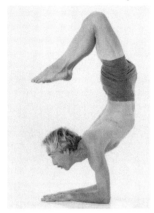

4. **Advanced** Students, balancing on your forearms, with slow deep breathing, bend your knees, lowering your feet toward the top of your head. Hold this for another three complete breaths. **Advanced** students can place legs in Lotus Posture for an additional three breaths. When finished, exhale and relax, lowering down into Child's Posture.

Crane and Sideways Crane (Bakasana)—*(Intermediate to Advanced)*

The word *baka* means "crane." In the initial variation of this posture, you resemble a crane wading in a quiet pond.

BENEFITS

The Crane is great for building your stomach, arm, and shoulder muscles. These postures will strengthen your wrists and improve your balance.

INSTRUCTIONS: TRANSITION FLOW

1. Start this posture from Child's Posture. Inhale, move your torso forward, and lift your torso upward into the Upward Facing Dog, then exhale, dropping your head and lifting your hips, as you move into the Downward Facing Dog.

2. From Downward Facing Dog, bend your elbows and knees, gently lowering your knees to touch the outside of your elbows. **Advanced** students can jump into Crane from Downward Facing Dog, engaging your *bandhas* and landing

softly on your elbows. If you have weak or troubled wrists, elevate the palms of your hands a few inches up off the floor with a yoga wedge or rolled towel. This will create less bend in the wrist and give better support.

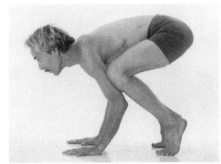

POSTURE FLOW

3. Spread your fingers wide for better support. Keeping your elbows bent, form a ledge to rest your knees on.

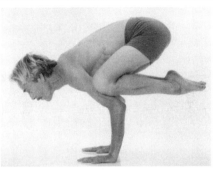

4. Lean your torso forward as you drop your head downward and take more of your body weight onto your elbows. Keep pushing gently forward with your toes and try to balance your knees on your elbows as you lift your feet off the floor. **Advanced** students try to straighten your arms, resting your knees in your armpits for an additional three breaths. **Beginners** relax into Child's Posture when finished. **Intermediate to advanced**: Jump back to Four Limbed Staff, then Upward Facing Dog, and relax into Child's Posture.

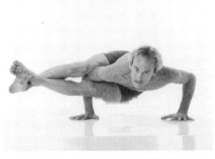

5. **Sideways Crane: Advanced** students follow Step I, then instead walk your feet and knees to your right side of your right elbow, keep your center of gravity low, and balance both knees and extended legs onto your right elbow, forming the Sideways Crane. Hold this position for five complete breaths, now move your right leg back behind you, extended into the air, for the Running Man Posture, for two more breaths. When finished, repeat on the opposite side. When finished, shake your wrists out and relax into the Child's Posture.

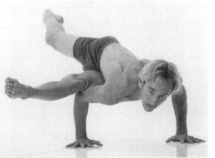

Handstand (Adho Mukha Vrksasana)—(Advanced)

The words *adho mukha* mean "facing downward," and *vrksa* means "tree." In this posture, you resemble an upside-down tree with its roots up in the air.

BENEFITS

The handstand builds strength and balance as it develops your chest and strengthens your shoulders, arms, and wrist. This posture is also a wonderful way to build your self-confidence.

INSTRUCTIONS: TRANSITION FLOW

Beginners and intermediate students can do this posture with the aid of a wall. First position your feet flat from a wall that is behind you.

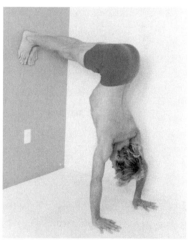

1. Start from the Child's Posture, inhale into Upward Facing Dog, then exhale into Downward Facing Dog Posture, resting on your hands and feet. **Beginners and intermediate**: Position your feet at the base of a wall which is behind you. Stabilize your balance and place one foot at a time on the wall, with legs parallel to the floor.

POSTURE FLOW

2. Keep your arms straight and balance, using the wall for support as you form a 90-degree angle with your torso. Practice lifting alternate legs up toward the ceiling, one at a time. Hold this pose for five complete breaths. When finished, exhale, lower your legs back to the ground, and relax into Child's Posture.

3. **Advanced:** If you are stable with your handstand, you can practice on your own, without the security of the wall. From Downward Facing Dog Posture as you inhale, you can jump into a handstand, or walk your feet closer to your hands. Now press your legs outward and up into a Handstand.

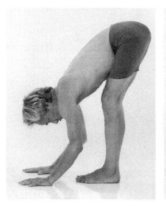
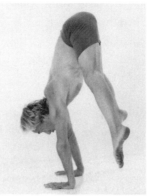
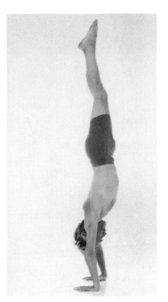

4. Strive to drop your head down and look out parallel to the floor, or close your eyes. Keep your spine straight and arms engaged, feel the energy from the Earth, and try to relax. Hold this posture for five to ten deep breaths, practice two repetitions then exhale, come down slowly, and relax into the Child's Posture.

5. **Upper Level Advanced** students can move from Handstand to Flying V Scale Posture Tolasana with straight legs toward ceiling, then take Muscle Power *vinyasa* to Four Limbed Staff, then to Upward Facing Dog, then to Downward Facing Dog, and Child's Posture.

Mountain Posture (Tadasana)—(All levels)

The Sanskrit word *tada* relates to a mountain, and in this posture you are taking on some of these characteristics by standing tall, strong, and grounded to the Earth's energy. There is no *vinyasa* with this posture, as this is a base posture contained within the *vinyasas*.

BENEFITS

The Mountain Posture helps to teach balance, correct posture, and self-confidence necessary to practice many of the yoga postures.

INSTRUCTIONS

1. Stand straight, relaxed, and firmly grounded with your feet together, spine straight, and shoulders back.

2. Allow your arms to hang relaxed by your sides, as you slightly pull your navel in toward your spine. Your vision is out parallel to the floor, and you are strong, yet relaxed and focused.

3. Hold this position for five complete breaths, when finished move on to your next posture or *vinyasa*.

Extended Triangle Posture (Utthita Trikonasana)—(*All levels*)

The word *utthita* means "extended" and *trikona* relates to a triangle. In this posture you will form an extended triangle with your body.

BENEFITS

This posture strengthens the muscles of your legs and creates more mobility in your hips. It will also stretch the sides of your torso, while teaching balance and coordination.

INSTRUCTIONS: TRANSITION FLOW

1.   Standing in Mountain Posture, take the Poetic Power Flow *vinyasa* (see page 146) to a wide stance, with your feet a little more than shoulder-width apart and your arms by your sides.

POSTURE FLOW

2.   On an inhalation, lift your arms up over your head, like an eagle stretching its wings. With your body weight evenly distributed between both feet, pivot your left foot outward toward your left. On an exhalation, lunge with your left leg, with your left arm in front of your torso and your right arm behind.

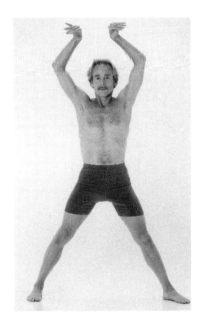
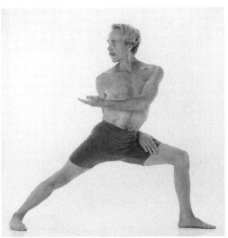

3. On an inhalation, straighten your leg and stretch your left arm outward to your left side, leaning to the left with your torso.

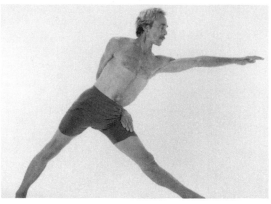

4. On an exhalation, make sure your left foot is pointing toward the left and pivot your right foot inward a bit less than 45 degrees. Try to keep your hips and shoulders open, on the same line as your torso. Continue your exhalation as you tilt your whole torso to your left side, lowering your left hand down, grabbing the big toe of your left foot. **Beginners**: If you are not particularly flexible, you can rest your left elbow on your left knee, or you can rest your left hand on a yoga block placed next to your left foot, outside your ankle.

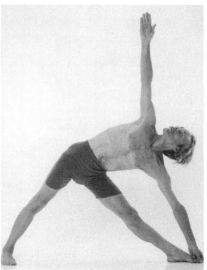

5. Place your right arm straight up into the air perpendicular to the floor, with your palm facing outward; you are gazing up at your hand. Your left hand is placed on the big toe of your left foot.

6. Begin doing your slow deep breathing. Keep your torso extended out over your right leg, try to keep your chest expanded, hips open, and your back flat. Turn your vision up toward your right hand as you gaze up toward the ceiling and lengthen your neck.

7. After holding this posture for five slow deep breaths, exhale all your air, and then, on the inhalation, lift your torso back to an upright standing position with your arms out in Eagle Wings. Then exhale and lower your arms down by your sides. Repeat the same exercise on the opposite side, then return to the Mountain Posture.

Twisted Extended Triangle Posture (Parivrtta Trikonasana)— (Intermediate)

Parivrtta means "twisted or revolved" and *trikona* is a "triangle." In this posture you will twist your torso around as you form an extended triangle.

BENEFITS

The Twisted Extended Triangle helps to relieve backaches, tones your spine, and strengthens your back. It helps to strengthen hamstring, thigh, and calf muscles.

INSTRUCTIONS: TRANSITION FLOW

Start by taking the Poetic Power Flow *vinyasa* (see page 146) to a wide stance, with your feet a little more than shoulder-width apart and your arms by your sides.

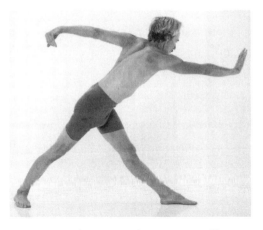

1. On an inhalation, lift your arms up parallel to the floor, then exhale, and lower your left arm down as you lift your right arm upward in a circular motion, like a windmill. Twist to the left side, pointing your left foot outward and pivoting your right foot in at 45-degree angle. Square off your torso and hips toward your left foot.

POSTURE FLOW

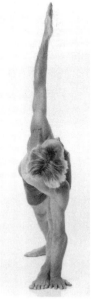

2. Lowering your right hand to the outside of your left foot, lift your left hand upward toward the ceiling, drawing one straight line from your supporting right hand through your shoulders and out your left fingertips. If you are not particularly flexible, just rest your right elbow onto your right knee, or rest your right hand on a yoga block.

3. Try to keep your hips squared and your torso extended out over your left supporting leg. Move your left hip back and your right shoulder under, lengthen through your neck, and keep your vision upward. Hold this posture for five complete breaths.

4. When finished, inhale and gracefully circle your extended arms as you return back to standing, then exhale, flowing down onto the opposite side, using the same technique.

5. When finished, inhale and return back to standing, lifting your arms up over your head, then relax and lower arms. With your arms by your sides, take the Poetic Power Vinyasa Flow back to the Mountain Posture.

Extended Side Angle Posture (Utthita Parsvakonasana) —(All levels)

Utthita means "stretched or extended," parsva means "side or flank," and kona relates to an "angle." In this posture you will form an extended side angle with your body.

BENEFITS

In the Extended Side Angle Posture you will strengthen legs and tone ankles, knees, and thighs. This posture can also help to develop your chest and reduce fat around your waist and abdominal area. This posture teaches a combination of strength and softness, grace and power.

INSTRUCTIONS: TRANSITION FLOW

1. Start with the Poetic Power Flow *vinyasa* to a standing position with both feet extended a little more than shoulder-width apart (see page 146). Stand with your knees slightly bent, torso upright, and imagine you are standing in the warm ocean water, as deep as your waist.

2. On an inhalation, move your right arm out across in front of your left leg, with your arm parallel to the floor, yet angled slightly downward and your elbow slightly bent, as if you were about to throw a Frisbee. Your left knee is bent, your left hand and arm is hanging down relaxed, behind your torso, yet at your left side of your body and angled slightly downward. On an inhalation, start bend-

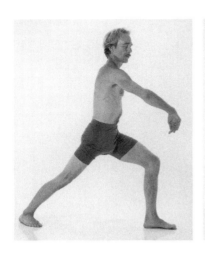 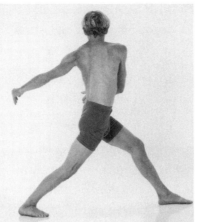 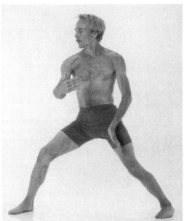

ing your body back to your right side, and visualize your left hand as if you were dragging this hand through the ocean water. Imagine that your right hand was throwing a Frisbee.

3. Continue your inhalation, moving the energy across in front of your body, as you start bending your right knee to your right side. Stand strong, yet relaxed, pivoting your right foot outward 90 degrees and pivoting your left foot in slightly at a 45-degree angle. Lifting your arms up to your right side with wrists soft, as you gaze to the right, start lunging deeper into your right knee.

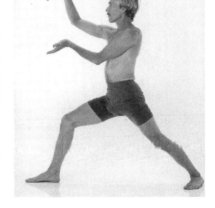

POSTURE FLOW

4. On an exhalation start the path to the floor. Lunge down onto your right leg forming a 90-degree angle with your right knee. Try to place your right hand softly on the outside of your right foot, resting onto the floor. If you are not quite that flexible, rest your elbow onto your knee, or

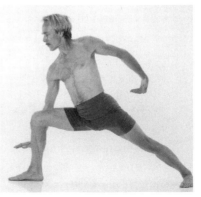

use a yoga block. Your left arm is extended above your head at a 45-degree angle, on the same plane as your torso.

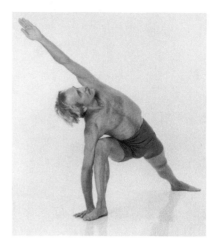

5. From your left extended foot through your torso and out your fingertips, you will form a nice 45-degree angle.

6. Turn your head upward, looking up toward the ceiling, trying to look up under your left arm and hold this position for five slow deep breaths. When you finish, on an inhalation, lift your left arm up, and repeat the same movement, this time moving to the left, drawing the energy across in front of your body, then exhale and lower yourself down to the left side for an additional five breaths. When finished, inhale and return smoothly to standing. Take Poetic Flow *vinyasa* back to standing, with feet together.

Twisted Extended Side Angle Posture (Parvritta Utthita Parsvakonasana)—(*Intermediate*)

Parvritta relates to being twisted, or turned around. *Utthita* means "stretched or extended," *parsva* means "side or flank," and *kona* relates to an "angle." In this posture you will form a twisted, extended side angle with your body.

BENEFITS

In the Twisted Extended Side Angle Posture you will strengthen legs and tone ankles, knees, and thighs. Your spine will be toned and invigorated. This posture can also help to develop your chest and reduce fat around your waist and abdominal area.

INSTRUCTIONS: TRANSITION FLOW

Begin with the Poetic Power Flow *vinyasa*, then follow the instructions below.

I. From a standing position with feet more than shoulder-width apart, right knee bent about 80 degrees, place both of your arms extended at your right side, just

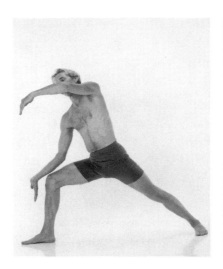
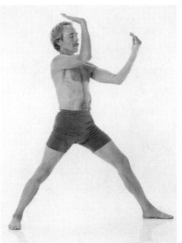

above your right thigh, as if you were holding a big beach ball, with hands and arms relaxed. On an inhalation, lift both arms in an arching motion, tracing a semicircle up in front of your body, from right to left.

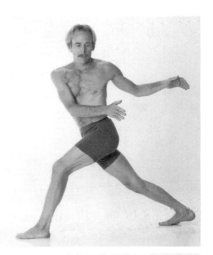

2. Draw a path with your left hand and follow with your right hand, keeping your wrist soft, as if you were moving under water. Continue your inhalation as you pivot your left foot outward about 90 degrees and your right foot inward about forty degrees. At the same time continue inhaling and twisting your torso to the left as you complete the arching motion of your arms, twisting to your left side and moving your hands and arms back behind your left hip, twisting your body in the same direction of energy.

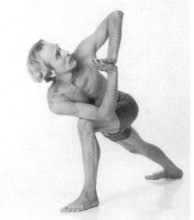

3. On an exhalation, lunge down deep on your left leg as you allow your hands to move together, with palms touching, in prayer fashion, and come softly to resting with your right elbow on your left thigh.

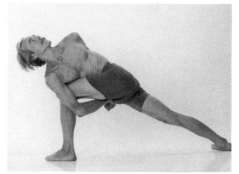

4. If your hips are not very flexible, you may come up on your right toes, taking some of the stretch out of your hip. If you are more flexible, strive to keep your right supporting foot flat on the ground. Try to form one line of energy from your right supporting leg through your torso and out the top of your head. Move your left hip back and your right shoulder under and keep your elbows expanded, away from one another. Hold this posture for five complete breaths. **Advanced** students try to grab your left wrist behind your back with your right hand.

5. When finished, on an inhalation begin to straighten your left leg, as you lift your arms in the same arching motion, leading with your right hand and following with your left. Repeat the same exercise instructions, only for your opposite side and when finished slowly flow back to standing, return through Poetic Power Flow to Mountain Posture and relax.

Expanded Foot Posture A-(Prasarita Padottanasana) —(All levels)

Pada means "foot" and *prasarita* means "spread, expanded, or extended." In this posture you will be stretching and moving energy in several different directions.

BENEFITS

This posture creates strength and flexibility in your hamstrings, calves, and ankles while bringing an easy blood supply to your torso and brain. The posture allows for more range of motion in your shoulders and also assists in creating an alternative for those who have not yet accomplished the Headstand.

INSTRUCTIONS: TRANSITION FLOW

Start from the Poetic Power Flow *vinyasa* (see page 146).

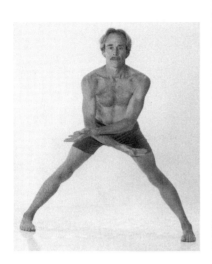 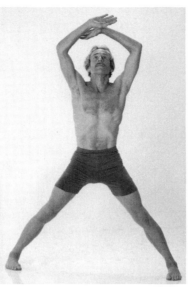 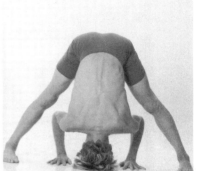

1. Stand with your spine straight and shoulders back, your feet slightly more than shoulder-width apart. Turn your toes slightly inward and heels outward, grounding yourself into the Earth with the outsides of your feet.

2. On an exhalation, cross your arms in front of your abdominal muscles. Lifting the energy upward, creating a circular motion as you lift your arms all the way up over your head. Now start your exhale, lowering your arms down, placing your hands between your expanded feet and trying to place your head down between your hands.

POSTURE FLOW

3. Place your wrist up under your elbows and make your arms parallel with one another. If you are more flexible, you can move your head back beyond the centerline of your torso. Keep your legs straight, unless you have tension in your lower back and legs, in which case you should bend your knees slightly, or place your hands on yoga blocks. Hold this position for five deep breaths.

4. When you are finished, lift your torso slowly, as you cross your arms in front of your body, in a circular motion, repeating Step 2, lifting the energy upward all the way up over your head, then exhale and lower your arms into the next variation.

Variations of this posture can be practiced by repeating Steps 1 and 2, then substituting the variations below for Step 3.

Variation 1 (**Intermediate**)—Interlacing your fingers, with arms extended behind your back, inhale as you arch backward, then exhale as you hinge forward at your waist lowering your head to the floor and your arms behind your back, opening your chest and shoulders. Hold this pose for five complete breaths.

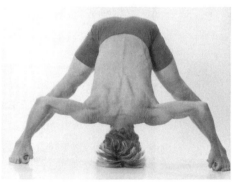

Variation 2 (**Intermediate**)—Inhale, lifting your arms up in a circular motion, then exhale, hinging forward at your waist, lowering your head to the floor as you reach down and grab the big toes of your extended feet. Hold this pose for five complete breaths.

Variation 3 (**Intermediate**)—Place your hands in prayer fashion behind your back. **Beginners** grab alternate elbows behind your back. Inhale as you arch backward, then exhale as you hinge forward at your waist, lowering your head to the floor and your arms behind your back, opening your chest and shoulders. Hold this posture for five complete breaths.

Variation 4 (**Intermediate**)—Place your hands in prayer fashion behind your back, as in Variation 3, only this time inhale as you twist your torso to the right side, then exhale and lunge forward on your right leg. You should balance solely on your right foot with your left leg extended behind you and your torso parallel to the

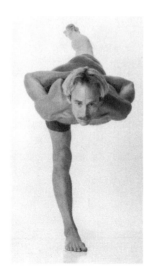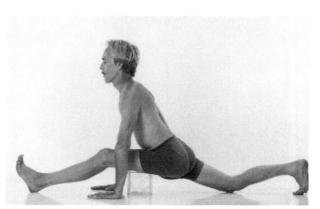

floor. Hold for three complete breaths, then return to the center and repeat on the opposite side. When finished return to standing and take Poetic Power Flow *vinyasa*.

Variation 5—(**Intermediate to Advanced**) Place your hands on the floor between your legs, then pivot your torso to the left, square your hips to the left, and split your legs to a comfortable stretch. **Intermediate** students can use a block for support up under your left hamstring muscle

Sundial Posture (Utthita Hasta Padangusthasana)— *(Intermediate)*

The word *utthita* means "extended," *hasta* means "hand," and *padangustha* relates to your big toe. In this posture you will extend your hand holding on to your big toe. I prefer to call this posture the Sundial, as you take a striking resemblance to this ancient clock.

BENEFITS

Teaches balance and posture, while strengthening your ankles, and muscles of your legs. Helps relieve stiff hips and firms abdominal muscles.

INSTRUCTIONS: TRANSITION FLOW

Begin in the Mountain Posture, with feet together and arms extended by your sides. Inhale, lifting your right arm forward and your left arm backward, sensing the energy around your body, moving with soft wrists, as if you were moving under water. Now exhale, lowering your arms back to your sides.

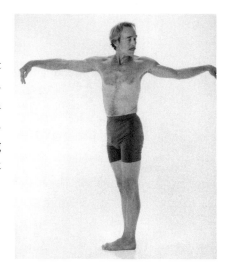

POSTURE FLOW

1. Exhale, lowering your arms, and place your left hand on your left hip as you bend your right leg, taking hold of your right big toe.

2. With your right hand, straighten your right leg, **beginners** keep knee bent, or hold knee instead of toes. Strive to keep your back straight and your hips squared. Hold this posture for five complete breaths. Now exhale and move your right leg to the right side of your body as you look to the left. Hold

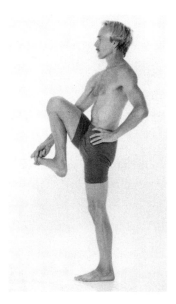 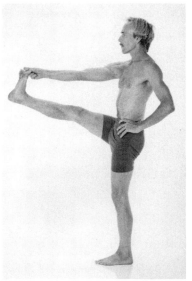 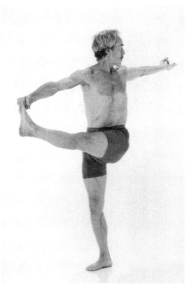

this posture for an additional three complete breaths. When finished, exhale and bring your right leg back to the center, then exhale and lower your leg to the floor. Repeat the same instructions, this time with your left leg extended. **Advanced** repeat the same instructions, only practice the twisted variation.

Warrior I and II (Virabhadrasana)—(All levels)

The Warrior Postures get their names from the powerful presence you embrace when practicing these strong *asanas*. In Hindu legend, this posture is dedicated to *Virabhadra*, the powerful hero created by *Siva* from his matted hair.

BENEFITS

Both postures tone and strengthen leg muscles, expand your chest, and help you develop deep, powerful breathing and good balance. They also relieve tension in your shoulders and back as well as strengthen your ankles.

INSTRUCTIONS

I. **Beginner's Transition**—Begin in Mountain Posture, with your feet together, standing strong. As you inhale, bend your knees and lift your arms out from the sides of your body, like an eagle stretching its wings, and expand your chest. At the same time, take a large step backward with your left leg

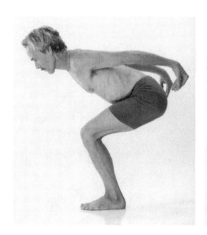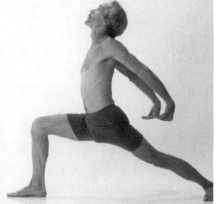

2. **Intermediate to Advanced Transition**—The entrance to this posture is through the full *vinyasa* movements of the Ultimate Power Sun Salutation. Follow the instructions for the Ultimate Power Salutation, only this time holding Warrior I for five complete breaths. When finished, open up to Warrior II for an additional five complete breaths. Make sure to practice both Warrior I and Warrior II on both sides.

WARRIOR I POSTURE—

1. Lunge down on your right leg with your knee over your heel and thigh parallel to the floor. Square your hips and shoulders forward toward your right foot, your arms are extended straight up over your head, with palms together and your gaze up toward your thumbs. If your shoulders and neck are very tight, leave your hands about one foot apart and gaze forward. Hold this position for five complete breaths. When finished, hold your deep, powerful stance and move on to the instructions for Warrior II.

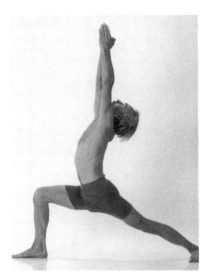

WARRIOR II POSTURE—

2. From Warrior I, open your hips, shoulders, and torso, right hip forward and left hip back. At the same time lower your arms down to rest parallel to the floor, on the same line as your torso, with palms facing downward.

3. Your right knee is still bent at 90 degrees with your knee over your heel. Lengthen through your fingertips in opposite directions. Your gaze should be forward parallel to the floor out over your right fingers. Stand very strong and yet relaxed, holding Warrior II for an additional five complete breaths.

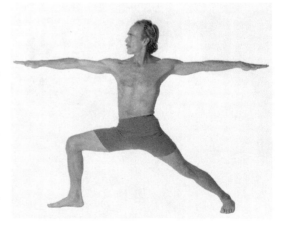

4. When finished, inhale, straighten your legs, and lift your torso back to the center, then exhale and flow down to Warrior I and II on the opposite side. Follow the same instructions only this time lunging with your left leg. When finished come back to standing and relax into Mountain Posture.

Warrior III Posture (Virabhadrasana)— (Intermediate to Advanced)

Warrior III is based within the same strong grounded standing posture as in Warrior I and II, only this time you will balance on one leg. This posture was named for the three avenues of energy flow: your arms point forward, one leg backward, and one leg as a supporting foot.

TRANSITION FLOW

Use the same transition flow as for Warrior I and Warrior II.

POSTURE FLOW

This is a difficult posture, so if you are a beginner, try positioning yourself in front of a wall, and as you balance on your supporting foot place your hands flat against the wall for support; this modification works quite well.

1. Start this posture from the Mountain Posture, standing with your spine straight and shoulders back and your feet together, arms resting by your sides.

2. Square your hips, shoulders, and torso in a forward position and plant your feet firmly on the ground. Inhale raising your arms up over your head, stretching your body long, with palms touching one another.

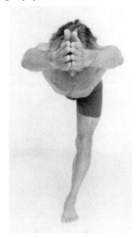

3. Now lean forward and balance all your weight onto your left leg; straighten your left leg and lift your right leg up off the floor, with your right leg extended behind you parallel to the floor. Your whole body should be balancing parallel to the floor, supported only by your left foot. Your arms extended out in front of you, with palms together and your gaze directed down toward the floor.

4. Hold this position for five slow deep breaths. When finished, on an exhalation, bend your left knee and slowly lower your right foot back to the floor, returning to the Mountain Posture and relax.

5. Repeat the same exercise, switching your balance to your right leg and extend your left leg behind you.

CATEGORY #9: DEEP RELAXATION POSTURES

Folded Leaf Posture—(All levels)

This posture is named the Folded Leaf because your body resembles a leaf, gently folded onto the soft grass. You can use Folded Leaf Posture as a counter-stretch between other yoga postures, or just as a nice way to relax in itself.

BENEFITS

In the Folded Leaf you will receive a gentle stretch on the entire length of your spine, create an easy flow of oxygenated blood to your brain, and achieve a very relaxing state of mind. If you are not very flexible and feel this variation is too difficult for you, try placing a pillow up under your hips and another under your chest, for support.

INSTRUCTIONS

1. Start by resting on your knees in the Thunderbolt Posture.

2. Lean forward, resting your torso on your thighs, with your forehead resting on the floor, arms extended by your sides, palms facing upward, toes pointed. If you have a problem with your knees, place a small pillow under your hips and a blanket up under your torso.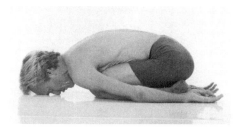

3. Maintain slow deep inhalations and exhalations. Energy flow is in a neutral posture; this means let your body channel energy from the Earth without directing the flow. Calm your mind and relax for five to ten breaths. When finished, inhale and return to Thunderbolt Posture.

Eye Exercise-(All levels)

In this posture you will exercise the eyes by moving them in various directions.

BENEFITS

Eye exercise strengthens the eyes, helps to enhance vision, and releases stress headaches.

INSTRUCTIONS

1. Sit quietly in your favorite seated posture, with good posture and with your eyes open, gazing forward.

2. Without moving your head, look as far up and then as far down as you can, three times each way. Now close your eyes and rest your palms of your hands over your eyes for a few seconds and relax.

3. Repeat the same exercise only this time looking as far to the right and back to the left as you can, without moving your head, three times each way. Then rest your hands over your eyes and relax once again.

4. Repeat one more time, but this time trace two full circles with your eyes in a clockwise direction and then again in a counterclockwise direction. Once again close your eyes and relax your hands over your eyes. When finished, lower your hands to your lap and sit quietly.

Stomach roll—(All levels)

In this posture you will learn to isolate your stomach muscles as you roll them from one side to the other.

BENEFITS

Stomach rolls can firm abdominal muscles and internal organs. They also release toxins from your intestinal tract.

1. From the Mountain Posture, stand with feet about shoulder-width apart, with knees bent and hands resting on your knees. Exhale all your air, squeezing it out with your abdominal muscles.

2. After you have completely exhaled, shift your weight from one side to the other by leaning slightly forward. At the same time try to loosen your stomach muscles, creating a rolling motion. You should look similar to a belly dancer. When finished, stand up and relax into the Mountain Posture.

Corpse Posture—(Svanasana)

In this posture, you will lay flat on your back and soak up the energy from the Earth.

BENEFITS

This relaxing posture helps to replenish the vital life force energy within your body, and creates a state of total deep relaxation. It also lowers blood pressure and releases stress and tension. Make sure you end every Sadhana Yoga practice with the Corpse Posture, or even better, the Deep Relaxation Exercise listed below.

INSTRUCTIONS

1. Lay down on your back with your feet about twelve inches apart, arms extended on the floor, by the sides of your body, with palms facing upward. Close your eyes and relax.

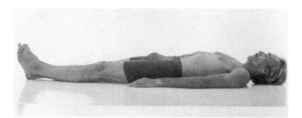

Deep Relaxation Exercise (All levels)

1. Begin in the Corpse Posture.

2. Lift your right leg about twelve inches from the floor, tense every muscle in your leg for a few seconds, then exhale, relax, and gently lower your leg to the floor. Repeat this step with your left leg.

3. Tighten the muscles in your hips and buttocks for a few seconds, and then exhale, relax, and let your gluteus muscles "melt" into the floor.

4. Arch your back, pressing down with your elbows and shoulders as you expand your chest toward the ceiling. Hold this posture for a few seconds, and then exhale, relax, and lower your back to the floor.

5. Press your lower back into the floor by tightening your buttock and stomach muscles as you press against the floor. Hold this posture for a few seconds, and then exhale and relax completely.

6. Lift your right arm about twelve inches off the floor, tensing all the muscles. Hold this posture for a few seconds, and then exhale, relax, and lower your arm to the floor. Repeat this step using your left arm.

7. Roll your head slowly to the right, and then to the left. Return your head to the center, exhale, and relax.

8. Fill your mouth with air, blowing your cheeks out like balloons. Hold for a couple of seconds, and then exhale, relax, and release the air.

9. Gently stretch all your facial muscles and then relax them. Close your eyes, take five slow, deep breaths, and clear your mind. Now go back once again and, working from your toes to your head, visualize each part of your body and mentally allow each muscle to relax, one by one, starting at your toes and working toward your head, relaxing on exhalations.

10. Now turn your focus internally, visualize your heart, exhale, and mentally ask your heart to relax. Visualize your brain, exhale, and calm it by releasing your thoughts as you calm and relax your mind.

11. Clear your mind of all but the most pleasant and positive thoughts. Visualize a beautiful place in nature and imagine yourself in this scene of beauty. Remain in this state of mind for five to fifteen minutes.

12. When you are finished, slowly stretch your arms over your head on an inhalation, then exhale and roll over onto your right side, with your arms and legs slightly bent. Remain in this position for a few breaths.

13. When you are finished, gradually return to a sitting position and try to preserve the positive uplifting thoughts that you created.

Vinyasas are the heart and soul of the Sadhana Yoga program. You use the *vinyasa* as a means of entering and exiting each yoga posture. These connecting movements prevent any break in the energy flow of your routine and create a smooth flowing grace. For example, if you are in a seated posture and you need to go into a standing posture, you can scramble to your feet, frantically tug at your workout clothes, and slowly with the grace of a drunken elephant, put yourself into the next position.

When you use a *vinyasa* to move from one posture to the next, you increase your body heat and *prana* energy, and you maintain the power of your routine's momentum. By doing your *vinyasa* right, you will take on the beauty and power of nature. Ignore them, and your routine is scattered, disconnected, and much less effective.

HOT AND COLD VINYASAS

In Sadhana Yoga there are two basic types of *vinyasas*. Each of these *vinyasas* has its own character and is appropriate for different phases of your practice. Some *vinyasas* need to be very strenuous in order generate body heat. These *vinyasas* demand more muscular work and are designed to be more active. I call these "hot *vinyasas*."

Other *vinyasas* are designed to be less demanding on your muscles and create less heat, yet they still build energy and power. These "cool *vinyasas*" are less strenuous movements between your yoga postures.

Every level of practice should include both hot and cool *vinyasas*. A wise *yogi* or *yogini* might plan on using the cooler *vinyasas* when you first begin practicing. As you become more experienced, you can incorporate the hotter *vinyasas* into your routines.

Using Sadhana Yoga with Other Styles of Yoga Practice

Traditionally, most *Hatha* Yoga practices discourage their students from combining elements of other yoga styles. Sadhana Yoga is a complete system in itself, and yet at the same time you can use these techniques to greatly enhance whatever style of yoga you may be practicing. To incorporate Sadhana Yoga into your regular style, simply practice your yoga postures as you usually do, and when finished use my unique *vinyasas* to transport you to the next posture.

SOFT TOUCH-COOL *VINYASA* I
(BEGINNER TO ADVANCED)—

This wonderful *vinyasa* is perfectly appropriate for both novice and expert Sadhana Yoga practitioners.

When to use this vinyasa:

Use this *vinyasa* anytime you want to move from a seated to a standing posture, or in reverse. You can always use this *vinyasa* as a transitional flow into a Shoulder Stand, or as a link between two seated postures. This *vinyasa* builds heat and *prana* energy, helps to distribute *prana* energy, and clears your energy for a new posture. This cooler *vinyasa* requires minimum amounts of energy.

BENEFITS

In this cooler *vinyasa*, you stretch and counter-stretch your back and neck, as you invigorate your spine with the movement's wave-like motion. This *vinyasa* teaches balance, grace, and self-confidence. The brain receives a gentle, peaceful vibration due to the *vinyasa's* gentle, fluid movement, and quiet transition.

INSTRUCTIONS (SOFT TOUCH I) *VINYASA*

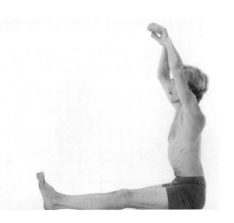

1. Start this *vinyasa* from the Seated Angle Posture, sitting on the floor with your legs extended straight in front of you and your arms resting on your extended legs.

2. On an inhalation, lift the energy upward, raising your arms with soft wrists, as you allow them to slide up your legs, and then up in front of your torso. Continue your inhalation as you lift the energy and your arms all the way up over your head.

3. Start your exhalation, and slowly bend your elbows, returning the energy to the Earth, lowering your arms down over your chest,

with hands placed together in prayer fashion. As you lower your arms, bend your knees and bring your feet in toward your torso.

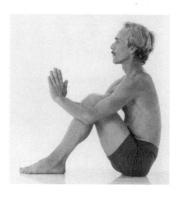

4. Continue exhaling, moving your weight onto your hands, and raising your hips from the floor while you roll your torso forward, dropping your head with your gaze on the floor in front of your toes. Continue exhaling, as you straighten your legs and flow into a Standing Forward Bend.

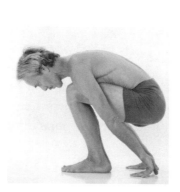 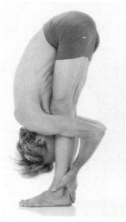

5. Inhale as you begin to lift your torso, bend your knees slightly as you create a wave lift motion with your body drawing the energy upward, as you lift your arms up in front of your torso, with wrists soft. Continue inhalation as you come to a full standing position and arch gently backward. Now exhale and lower your hands down over your chest, bringing the energy to rest in your torso, as you return your hands back to your sides into Mountain Posture. This would complete your transition to standing postures.

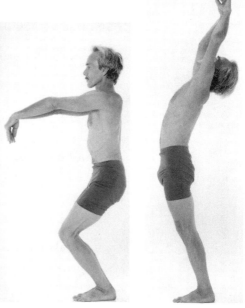

If you desire to take the full *vinyasa* back to sitting, or if you started from standing and wish to transition into a seated posture, continue with these instructions.

6. On an inhalation, lift the energy upward as you raise your arms up over your head, coming to a full standing position and arch gently backward.

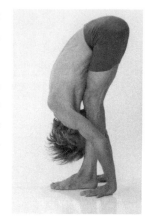

7. On an exhalation, slowly hinge forward at your waist, moving the energy toward the Earth, as you flow into your Standing Forward Bend, placing your hands on the floor beside your feet. If you find this stretch too intense, try keeping your knees slightly bent and lower your hands to your chin, rather than the floor, or you can place your hands onto some yoga blocks.

8. Inhale bending your knees, lowering your hips toward the floor, as if your were going to sit into a chair. At the same time, lifting your arms up parallel to the floor, as if your were a ski racer. On an exhalation, lower your hands down toward the floor. Continue the exhalation placing your hands on the floor beside your hips. Finish your *vinyasa* by straightening your legs, as you softly sit down on the floor into a Seated Angle Posture and relax.

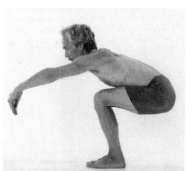
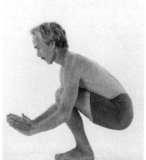
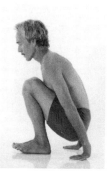
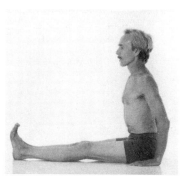

POETIC POWER FLOW-*VINYASA* #2:

The Standing Transition Jump-(Beginner-Advanced)—

When you practice Poetic Power Flow *vinyasa*, you look like an eagle stretching its wings before flight. Both beginning and more advanced Sadhana Yoga students use this cooler *vinyasa*. This *vinyasa* maintains moderate body heat and creates a soothing poetic flow between yoga postures. At the same time it creates enormous power and energy.

When to use this vinyasa:

Use this *vinyasa* anytime you want to move from one standing posture to another, or to connect a series of standing postures.

BENEFITS

The Standing Transition Jump enhances your energy flow, builds strength, and creates a focused mind. It also strengthens your ankles and leg muscles and teaches you to combine softness with power in your Sadhana Yoga program. This *vinyasa* also can improve your balance, rhythm, and coordination, and over a period of time it can open up tight shoulders and help relieve tension.

INSTRUCTIONS

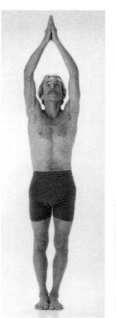
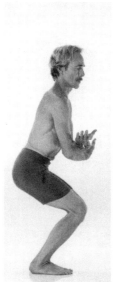

1. Start from Mountain Posture, with your feet together and your arms extended at your sides, with good posture. On an inhalation, move the energy upward by starting to lift your arms up over your head. Keep your wrists soft and relaxed as you lift your arms all the way up over your head, palms touching.

2. On an exhalation, lower your arms and cross them in front of your body, drawing the energy into your torso, at the same time bending your knees, as if you were getting ready to jump.

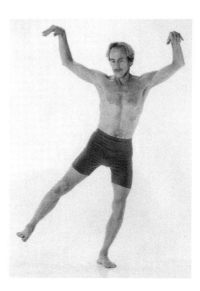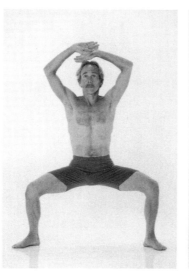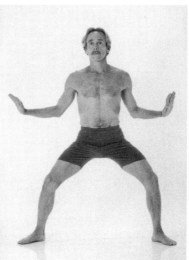

3. Start your inhalation and step, or jump 90 degrees to your right side, as you lift the energy up over your head, lifting your arms out and upward, landing in a wide stance, to your right side, with your feet more than shoulder-width apart. As you land, bend your knees deeply to absorb the shock. Your arms should now be up over your head, with palms facing outward and elbows bent.

4. As soon as you land, start your exhalation and begin to straighten your legs as you move the energy off to the sides of your body, by lowering your arms down to your sides. Straighten your legs and lower arms to your sides and relax. You are now ready to move into your standing posture.

After you finish your standing posture, repeat these steps, only in reverse, as you step or jump back to a forward-facing standing position. You will end in the Mountain Posture.

MUSCLE POWER-HOT *VINYASA* #3
(INTERMEDIATE TO ADVANCED)—

This *vinyasa* is a more physically demanding link, appropriate for intermediate to advanced students. This link is used to connect any seated postures, or can be modified to take you all the way to standing and back.

BENEFITS

This *vinyasa* builds inner heat, strength, endurance, and stamina, and it stretches out the muscles of your back, chest, legs, and arms. Alternate this *vinyasa* with the cooler, or less strenuous variety for best overall results. For best success engage both your *mula bandha* and *uddiyana bandha* when practicing this *vinyasa*.

INSTRUCTIONS

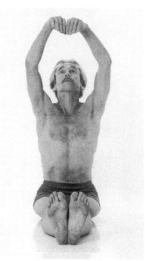

1. Start from the Seated Angle Posture, sitting upright on the floor with your legs extended out in front of your torso and your hands resting on your thighs. On an inhalation, gracefully raise the energy lifting your extended arms up in front and over your head, with soft wrists, as if you were moving under water.

2. When your arms are up overhead, exhale, lower your hands down in prayer fashion over your chest, as you bend your knees. Place your hands on the floor by your

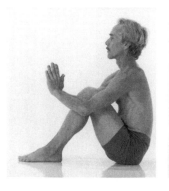
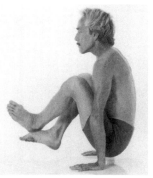

hips and on an inhalation, gather strength from the Earth, engage *mula* and *uddiyana bandhas*, as you push down with your hands, lifting your hips up off the floor. **Beginner to intermediate** students try placing a pair of yoga blocks under your hands as props in order to give you more extension, or roll forward onto your bent knees, with hips on the floor.

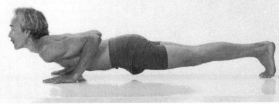

3. Pivot your torso, dropping your head downward, lifting your hips, as you push off from gravity and jump your legs backward, landing into Four Limb Staff Posture, exhale as you land, supported by your hands and feet only, resting about one inch off the floor.

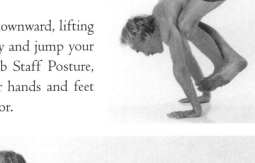

4. On an inhalation, lift the energy upward as you raise your torso upward and forward into the Upward Facing Dog Posture. Your torso arched, your chest expanded, and your gaze directed toward the sky supported totally on the tops of your feet and palms of your hands, keep your buttocks muscles engaged to avoid pressure on your low back.

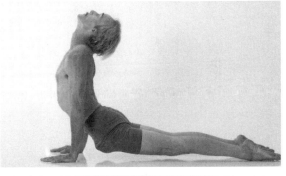

5. On an exhalation, drop your head down and lift your hips into the air forming a nice 90-degree angle with your body, resting on the bottoms of your feet. Strive to lower your heels to the floor. This is Downward Facing Dog.

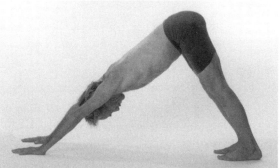

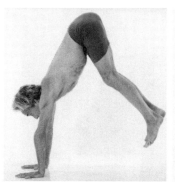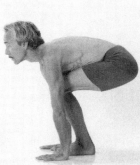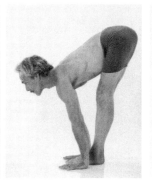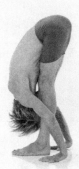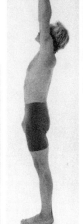

6. **For a transition to a seated position:** From Downward Facing Dog, lift your head looking up, between your hands, gathering strength, bending your knees and inhale, as you try to step, or jump your legs forward up beyond your hands, as you land softly into a Seated Angle Posture. **Beginner** students use a pair of yoga blocks up under your hands to allow for greater extension, or just step forward one foot at a time into the Seated Angle.

7. **For a transition to standing position:** On an inhalation, jump (or step for a lighter workout) your feet back between your hands and exhale when you land bending your knees. Inhale with hands remaining on the floor as you gaze upward, expanding your chest. Exhale as you move into the Standing Forward Bend. On an inhalation, lift your torso upward, pulling your arms out to your sides and up over your head, as you expand your chest, and stand with arms over head. Exhale and relax into the Mountain Posture.

8. If you are in a standing posture and want to transcend to a seated posture, simply follow the instructions in reverse.

Yoga posture practice is the ultimate physical and mental discipline. As you become more comfortable with your practice, remember to be gentle and loving to yourself, and strive to maintain a peaceful, spiritual element within your yoga practice. Be noncompetitive and set a goal to build a personal practice which best suits your own ability and needs.

PRACTICING THE
BEGINNER PROGRAM

True enlightenment is found
Within realizing
You will always be a student

When you first start practicing Sadhana Yoga, you should not expect to master the whole system in one session. Be patient with yourself. Even if you plan on becoming a yoga teacher, always consider yourself a student first. In the beginning you may have times when you feel awkward, clumsy, humbled, and even frustrated. However, you will also have many moments where you feel comfortable, relaxed, and at home with this system.

Remember to enjoy the journey and try to look forward to your practice. The object is not to achieve the most advanced posture, it is to connect with the natural flow of energy, feel good about yourself, and develop inner peace. In the beginning it is a good idea to rest between your postures, whenever you feel it is necessary. In time you will create a continuous flow of practice. Gradually incorporate a better diet and try to feel the connection between all energy as you become a part of the flow.

Upon completing your very first yoga session, your mind and thoughts will be blessed with a soothing touch and a sense of inner peace will prevail. After a few weeks your body will start to become stronger and more flexible, and your attention span will increase while your stress level will decrease.

After four to six months of practice, you will have a whole new outlook on life. Your overall health will have increased dramatically. You will have a close bond with nature and find your personal energy, both physical and mental, to be in abundance. Your muscles will have more shape and tone as you lose weight and strengthen your body.

Two Steps Forward

In the beginning you will find times when it seems as if your yoga is not progressing. You might have sore muscles, or feel as if you are dragging yourself through the routine. These physical reactions are often signs for you to back off and quit trying so hard. You might want to switch to another activity so that you can cross-train, and minimize your time with yoga for a short while. Once you stop trying to push yourself, then you will realize that you are progressing nicely once again.

Before You Begin

Yoga clothes should be nonrestrictive, comfortable, and appropriate for your practice environment. As a beginning student, you might want to use some of the props mentioned in Chapter 4 during your yoga practice, including straps, blocks, and a small pillow. It is always a good idea to have a clean towel and a water bottle handy. I do not think any props should be absolute, and as you progress, the use of props should diminish somewhat, although at any level some props can be very helpful.

Yoga Postures and *Vinyasa* Practice

As a beginner, you should start practicing about two or three times each week, with each session being anywhere from 45 minutes to 1½ hours. After a few weeks to a month of practice you can add more sessions per week and longer practice lengths. You will be ready to progress to the intermediate level when you feel comfortable with your present level of practice and are not worn out by the long routine. You can always give an intermediate routine a try and see how you feel afterward.

It is a good idea to become familiar with the individual yoga postures before you add all the flowing links. After a few weeks of practicing yoga, try adding a few *vinyasas* between your postures. After one or two months you should try to connect all your postures together with *vinyasas*.

Hard and Soft Flow Yoga

The type of *vinyasa* you choose to connect your postures together determines whether your yoga practice is Hard Flow or Soft Flow. The hot *vinyasa* (more strenuous) builds a Hard Flow workout, and cool *vinyasa* (less strenuous), creates a Soft Flow workout. For example, if you are practicing a very strenuous yoga posture and your entrance and exit are made of soft *vinyasas*, then your routine is considered to be Soft Flow. On the other hand, if you are practicing very easy yoga postures and connecting them with physically strenuous *vinyasas*, then this practice would be considered Hard Flow.

The yoga posture instructions each come with suggestions for a matching *vinyasa*. You can choose to incorporate that particular *vinyasa*, or choose another from those listed at the end of Chapter 4.

YOGA SEQUENCING

Yoga sequencing is designed to enhance your whole body physically and mentally. It is important for you to follow the proper order of yoga postures as laid out in the routines I have provided. If you randomly choose any yoga posture and disregard the proper sequencing, you will have a much greater risk of injury, lose connection with the energy flow, and become tired and unfocused after the practice.

INSTRUCTIONS FOR THE ROUTINES

The two workout routines listed in this chapter are presented as either short or long, depending on how much time you have to practice. The length of time given for each routine is only a general guideline: remember that you should never rush your routine. Yoga is best when you take your time.

If you choose the long routine and then find that you do not have enough time to finish, the next time you can start where you left off. However, always start your routine with breathing and yoga warm-ups, then add the postures, and finish with cool-down exercises, more breathing, and deep relaxation. So, if you only get halfway through your routine and time does not allow you to finish, make sure to finish with your deep relaxation, and at the next practice start with breathing, warm-ups, and then return to where you left off the previous session.

Instructions for Sitting and Breathing

Seated postures are a great way to begin practicing yoga breathing techniques. You can choose from any of the seated yoga postures, although most beginning students find the Perfect Posture to be comfortable and relaxing. For a more holistic approach, try a different seated posture at each different practice sessions.

HINTS AND SUGGESTIONS FOR BEGINNERS:

- *If your hips are tight and your leg muscles are not flexible, try placing a small pillow under your hips, and if necessary, under your knees as well.*
- *Strive to create good posture with your shoulders back and spine straight. Take your time: relax and enjoy the soothing touch of energy.*
- *Remember that exhalation is just as important as inhalation, so make the effort to completely empty your lungs before each inhalation.*
- *Draw energy into your body on inhalations and release stress and tension on exhalations.*
- *Review Chapter 3 for complete details on yoga breathing. You will find the seated-posture variations and instructions listed in Chapter 4.*

Yoga Warm-up Exercises

Always take time to warm up and try be kind to your body. Warm-up exercises are a important step to a fulfilling yoga practice, so don't skip these wonderful exercises in order to save time.

Inverted Yoga Postures-Hints and Suggestions for Beginners

The most difficult yoga postures are the inverted postures, which are very energizing and create a nice tranquil flow for your practice. Beginners should place a folded towel under your shoulders in the Shoulder Stand to help create more comfort and avoid injury. Both the Fish and Bridge Postures are counter-stretches for the Shoulder Stand: you should always practice one or the other after completing a Shoulder Stand. If you have a problem or injury in your neck, then you would find the Bridge Posture more comfortable than the Shoulder Stand. If you have an injury to your neck, avoid practicing the Headstand Posture.

Inverted postures should be avoided if you have any of the following physical conditions:

- *a floating retina*
- *during your menstrual cycle*
- *severe injury to your neck*
- *glaucoma*
- *extreme high blood pressure*

DEEP RELAXATION (5–10 MINUTES):

As a beginner student you should understand the true value of this relaxation exercise. Always save time for relaxation: it helps to replenish the vital life-force energy within your body and creates a state of total deep relaxation. Make sure you end every Sadhana Yoga practice with the Corpse Posture, or better yet the deep relaxation exercise on page 116.

BEGINNER SHORT ROUTINE:
(40–50 MINUTE PRACTICE)

Practice the following routine by completing each of the exercises and postures listed. Pay attention to the durations for each posture, and strive to hold each posture for the duration given.

Perfect Posture	(See pg 53)
Yoga Breathing	(See pg 37)

YOGA WARM-UPS

Alternate the Cat Stretch during your first session, and the Sun Salutation at your next session.

Neck rolls and Shoulder rolls	(See pg 58, 59)
Cat Stretch (two repetitions)	(See pg 64)
Soft Touch *Vinyasa* I (upward)	(See pg 143)
Soothing Touch–Sun Salutation (two repetitions)	(See pg 66)

STANDING POSTURES

Alternate Triangle Posture at one practice session and the Twisted Triangle at the next.

Extended Triangle Posture	(see pg. 123)
Twisted Extended Triangle	(see pg. 125)
Soft Touch *Vinyasa* I (downward)	(see pg. 143)

INVERSIONS AND COUNTER-STRETCHES

Shoulder Stand	(see pg. 81)
Bridge Posture as Counter-Stretch	(see pg. 84)

Remember to breathe as you are stretching, exhale, release stress and tension as you move slightly deeper into your stretch, inhale embracing energy as you back off from the stretch slightly.

Staff Posture	(see pg. 87)
Seated Forward Bend	(see pg. 88)
Head Knee Posture (A)	(see pg. 91)

BACK BENDS

Cobra	(see pg. 100)
Bow	(see pg. 104)

SPINAL TWIST

Spine Toner	(see pg. 109)

DEEP RELAXATION

Corpse Posture and deep relaxation exercise	(see pg. 140)

Beginner Long Routine (1 hour to 1:30 minute practice)

Practice the following routine by completing each of the exercises and postures listed. Pay attention to the durations for each posture, and strive to hold each posture for the duration given. If you find you do not have enough time to complete this routine in your allotted amount of time, simply skip ahead to the relaxation exercise and then finish the last half of your practice the next session.

SEATED POSTURES AND YOGA BREATHING

Perfect Posture	(See Page 53)
Yoga Breathing (10 breaths)	(See Page 37)

YOGA WARM-UP EXERCISES

Perform all three of the postures listed, in order of sequence.

Neck rolls and Shoulder rolls	(see pg. 58, 59)
Cat Stretch (two repetitions)	(See Page 64)
Soft Touch *Vinyasa* I (upward)	(see pg. 143)
Sun Salutation–Soothing Touch (four repetitions)	(See Page 66)

STANDING POSTURES

Perform all three of the postures listed, in order of sequence.

Extended Triangle Posture	(See Page 123)
Twisted Triangle Posture	(See Page 125)
Extended Side Angle Posture	(See Page 126)
Soft Touch *Vinyasa* I (downward)	(see pg. 143)

INVERSIONS AND COUNTER-STRETCHES

Perform all three of the postures listed, in order of sequence.

Shoulder Stand	(See Page 81)
Fish	(See Page 85)
Bridge	(See Page 84)

LEG STRETCHES

Perform all three of the postures listed, in order of sequence.

Staff	(See pg. 87)
Seated Forward Bend	(See Page 88)
Head Knee Posture (A)	(See Page 91)
Seated Angle Posture	(See Page 93)

BACK-BEND POSTURES

Perform all three of the postures listed, in order of sequence.

Cobra	(See Page 100)
Full Locust	(See Page 103)
Bow	(See Page 104)

SPINAL TWISTING POSTURES

Twist Posture I	(See Page 109)

DEEP RELAXATION (5–20 MINUTES)

PRACTICING THE
INTERMEDIATE PROGRAM

One brief moment

Of practice

Is worth more than a millennium

Of thought

Intermediate students have acquired some degree of self-confidence and have tasted many

of yoga's physical benefits. This background will work to your advantage as you incorpo-

rate the lessons of Sadhana Yoga into your yoga practice.

Intermediate students should feel free to practice any of the beginner-level routines

as an alternative to the routines listed in this section. Just as with a beginner practice,

don't be intimidated by thumbing ahead to the more extreme postures. There is no evidence to support the notion that those practicing advanced-level postures are any more spiritual, wise, or enlightened than those at the intermediate level. The Buddha once said: "The path to enlightenment is the middle line." It is much more important to have a comfortable, quality practice than to push yourself beyond your current limits and not enjoy the routine.

Lessons for the Intermediate Student

Environment: As an intermediate student, you can begin to think about practicing outdoors at least twice a month, weather permitting. Ideally the temperature should be moderate and comfortable, whatever that means to you. As a intermediate student, you should strive to find comfort in all situations and make the best of what you have to work with.

Props: Although you are an intermediate student, you still might want to use straps and blocks, and a small pillow as needed. You might also want to have a clean towel and a bottle of filtered water handy.

Remember that the main object of Sadhana Yoga is to connect with the natural flow of energy. As an intermediate student, it is a good idea to connect more of your postures together with *vinyasas* and rest between your postures less, only when you feel it is necessary. In time strive toward having a continuous flow of practice.

As an intermediate student, you will find that yoga is starting to touch your soul in a positive way. Your mind will be more focused and you will feel almost anything is possible. This mind focus will branch out in to your daily life and assist you in every aspect of your existence.

Should I skip certain postures which are very difficult for me?

Postures which are very difficult are usually the ones you need to practice more. You can master the harder postures by beginning to practice the preliminary steps of each one. Once you can get each piece right, the next step is to try the easier variations of hard-to-achieve postures. You'll find that you will quickly get the hang of every posture.

Moving Forward

As an intermediate student it is often good to go back and practice some routines from the beginner-level workout. This will give you the opportunity to concentrate on developing a nice flow with a less-demanding yoga workout. Then you can carry these concepts of flow with some newfound self-confidence into your intermediate-level practice. I first discovered the concept of "softness is strength" by holding on to a beautiful soft-flowing line of energy in a less intimidating routine, then carrying it with me to a more advanced workout.

YOGA POSTURES AND *VINYASA*

As an intermediate-level student, you should be practicing about three or four times each week, with a session lasting anywhere from 50 minutes to 1½ hours. After a month of practice you can add more sessions per week and longer practice lengths. You should also pick a week to cross-train up and down the levels of yoga practice, picking more strenuous routines one day, light ones the next, or pick another day and do less postures, yet hold them longer, and the following day have a casual outdoor practice.

As an intermediate student, you are ready to experience the benefits of the *vinyasas*. Try adding all your *vinyasas* between yoga postures, creating a wonderful flow to your practice. After a month you should try to focus on recognizing the energy flow you feel when moving between your postures. You can try to connect with this energy and set it down gently as you enter your posture.

HARD AND SOFT FLOW YOGA

The type of *vinyasa* you choose to connect your postures determines whether your yoga practice is Hard Flow or Soft Flow. The hot *vinyasa* (more strenuous) builds a Hard Flow workout, and cool *vinyasa* (less strenuous), which creates a Soft Flow workout. For example, if you are practicing a very strenuous yoga posture and your entrance and exit are made of soft *vinyasas*, then your routine is considered to be Soft Flow. On the other hand, if you are practicing very easy yoga postures and connecting them with physically strenuous *vinyasas*, then this practice would be considered Hard Flow.

The *vinyasas* for each separate posture are located with the posture instructions, labeled as "transition flow." You can choose to incorporate this *vinyasa* or choose another from those listed at the end of Chapter 4.

YOGA SEQUENCING

Yoga sequencing is designed to enhance your whole body physically and mentally. It is important for you to follow the proper order of yoga postures as laid out in the routines I have provided. If you randomly choose any yoga posture and disregard the proper sequencing, you will have a much greater risk of injury, lose connection with the energy flow, and become tired and unfocused after the practice.

INSTRUCTIONS FOR THE ROUTINES

The two workout routines listed in this chapter are presented as either short or long, depending on how much time you have to practice. The length of time given for each routine are only general guidelines: remember that you should never rush your routine; yoga is best when you take your time.

If you choose the long routine and then find that you do not have enough time to finish, the next time you can just start where you left off. However, always start your routine with breathing and yoga warm-ups, then add the postures, and finish with cool-down exercises, more breathing, and deep relaxation. So, if you only get halfway through your routine and time does not allow you to finish, make sure to finish with your deep relaxation, and at the next practice start with breathing, warm-ups, and then return to where you left off the day before.

INSTRUCTIONS FOR SITTING AND BREATHING

As a intermediate student you should try to refine your breathing techniques, expanding inhalations and exhalations. Rotate the different seated postures through your practice routines, choosing a different one in separate practice sessions.

HINTS AND SUGGESTIONS FOR INTERMEDIATE STUDENTS:

- *As an intermediate student, challenge yourself by holding your seated postures a bit longer. If your hips are very tight and leg muscles nonflexible, try placing a small pillow under your hips, and if necessary, under your knees as well.*
- *Strive to create good posture as you visualize a beautiful nature scene with your shoulders back and spine straight.*
- *Remember that exhalation is just as important as inhalation, so make the effort to completely empty your lungs before each inhalation.*
- *Draw energy into your body on inhalations and release stress and tension on exhalations.*
- *Test yourself on the breathing techniques in Chapter 3 and try to use these techniques on and off the yoga mat.*

At the intermediate-level, warm-ups are still a very important aspect of your practice. Always take time to warm up and try to be kind to your body. Warm-up exercises are an important step to fulfilling your enhanced endurance and aerobic qualities within yoga practice, so don't skip these wonderful exercises in order to save time.

Sun Salutation Information

In this level routine you will notice I have added two separate Sun Salutations. You can alternate between the two at separate practice sessions, or practice two repetitions of each. All the Sun Salutations in this program are very beneficial for intermediate level students and you should try to incorporate the variety into your ongoing practice.

STANDING POSTURES

The standing postures in the intermediate level routines are connected with *vinyasas*. Once every few weeks you should close your eyes during your standing postures in order to enhance balance and get in touch with the Earth energy.

INVERSIONS AND COUNTER-STRETCHES

The most difficult yoga postures are the inverted postures, which are very energizing and create a nice tranquil flow for your practice. Unless you are very experienced, it is a good idea to place a folded towel under your shoulders in the Shoulder Stand, in order to help create more comfort and avoid injury. Both the Fish and Bridge postures are counterstretches for the Shoulder Stand: you should always practice one or the other after completing a Shoulder Stand. If you have a problem or injury in your neck, then you would find the Bridge Posture more comfortable.

There are also some circumstances when you should check with your doctor before attempting inverted postures. Inverted postures should be avoided if you have any of the following physical conditions:

- *a floating retina*
- *during your menstrual cycle*
- *severe injury to your neck*
- *glaucoma*
- *extreme high blood pressure*

LEG STRETCHES

At the intermediate level these leg stretches will serve as a great stepping-stone to assist you in other postures in higher level practice. Start to move deeper into your leg stretches, and once a week hold them for twice the breath count. Listen to your body and respect your limits. If you should pull or strain a muscle in practice, by all means back off, give these postures a rest, and try to cross-train with other physical activities.

ARM BALANCE POSTURES

The arm balance postures can be quite challenging, and you will receive quite an anaerobic workout from lifting your own body weight. As you attempt these, remember to spread your fingers wide for better stability.

DEEP RELAXATION (5–20 MINUTES)

As an intermediate student, you should understand the true value of this relaxation exercise. Always save time for relaxation: it helps to replenish the vital life force energy within your body, and creates a state of total deep relaxation. Make sure you end every Sadhana Yoga practice with the Corpse Posture, or better yet the deep relaxation exercise in Chapter 4.

Intermediate Short Routine: (45–60 minutes)

SEATED POSTURES AND YOGA BREATHING

Perfect Posture or Lotus Posture	(see pg. 53)
Yoga Breathing (10 complete breaths):	(see pg. 37)

YOGA WARM-UPS

Perform each of the following postures in the order they are listed.

Neck rolls and Shoulder rolls	(see pg. 58, 59)
Cat Stretch (two repetitions)	(see pg. 64)
Soft Touch *Vinyasa* I (upward)	(see pg. 143)
Sun Salutation–Soothing Touch Level #1 (Two Repetitions)	(see pg. 66)

STANDING POSTURES

Perform each of the following postures in the order they are listed.

Twisted Extended Triangle	(see pg. 123)
Warrior I	(see pg. 135)

INVERSIONS AND COUNTER-STRETCHES

In the intermediate practice you will find both Headstand and Shoulder Stand postures, try to keep your spine straight, drawing one line, which creates a stronger posture.

Soft Touch *Vinyasa* I (downward)	(see pg. 143)
Shoulder Stand	(see pg. 81)
Headstand	(see pg. 77)
Fish or Bridge (Counter Stretch)	(see pg. 84 or 85)

Perform each of the following postures in the order they are listed.

Staff Posture	(see pg. 87)
Seated Forward Bend	(see pg. 88)

BACK BENDS

Perform each of the following postures in the order they are listed.

Cobra	(see pg. 100)
Full Locust	(see pg. 103)

SPINAL TWIST

Twist Posture I	(see pg. 109)

ARM BALANCE

Crane Posture	(See Page 118)

DEEP RELAXATION

Always take the time for a quality deep relaxation. Some students find it helpful to use an eye pillow and light background music.

Corpse Posture–Deep relaxation (5–20 minutes)	(see pg. 140)

Intermediate Long Routine (1 hour to 1:30 minute practice)

If you find you do not have enough time to complete this routine, simply take relaxation and finish the last half of your practice the next session.

SITTING AND BREATHING

Perfect Posture or Lotus	(See Page 53)
Yoga Breathing (10 breaths)	(See Page 37)

YOGA WARM-UP EXERCISES

Please complete each of the following postures in the order as listed.

Neck rolls and Shoulder rolls	(see pg. 58, 59)
Cat Stretch (two repetitions)	(See Page 64)
Soft Touch *Vinyasa* I (upward)	(see pg. 143)
Willow Tree	(See Page 63)
Sun Salutation—Soothing Touch (four repetitions)	(See Page 66)
Sun Salutation—Ultimate Power (two repetitions)	(See Page 71)

STANDING POSTURES

Please complete each of the following postures in the order as listed.

Extended Triangle Posture	(See Page 123)
Twisted Extended Triangle Posture	(See Page 125)
Extended Side Angle Posture	(See Page 126)
Expanded Foot Posture	(See Page 130)
Warrior I	(See Page 135)
Muscle Power *Vinyasa* 3 (downward)	(see pg. 148)

Please complete each of the following postures in the order as listed.

Headstand	(See Page 76)
Fish	(See Page 85)
Shoulder Stand	(See Page 81)
Bridge	(See Page 84)

LEG STRETCHES

Please complete each of the following postures in the order as listed.

Staff	(see pg. 87)
Seated Forward Bend	(See Page 88)
Incline Plane	(See Page 90)
Head Knee Posture	(See Page 91)
Shooting the Bow (optional)	(See Page 97)

BACK BEND POSTURES

Please complete each of the following postures in the order as listed.

Cobra (3 repetitions)	(See Page 100)
Full Locust	(See Page 103)
Bow	(See Page 104)

Please complete each of the following postures in the order as listed.

Twist Posture I	(See Page 109)
Noose Posture	(See Page 111)

ARM BALANCE POSTURES

Please complete each of the following postures in the order as listed.

Scale	(See Page 116)
Crane	(See Page 118)
Sideways Crane	(See Page 119)

BREATHING AND PRANAYAMA

Lion Breathing Exercise (3 Repetitions)	(See Page 42)
Alternate Breathing (2 repetitions)	(See Page 41)

DEEP RELAXATION

Some students find it helpful to use an eye pillow and light background music.

Corpse Posture—Deep relaxation (5–20 minutes)	(see pg. 140)

PRACTICING THE
ADVANCED PROGRAM

Seek yoga to soften

The jagged stone

And touch the thoughts

That stand alone

Advanced students should strive not only to master the physical skills, but to achieve a

spiritual quality within their practice. Make an effort to maintain a full body-mind con-

nection, even during the most difficult routines. Keep peace and compassion in your

heart, be noncompetitive, and always take time to help the newcomer. Remember you

were once a beginner as well.

Lessons for Advanced Students

Be comfortable—The harder the yoga posture is, the more important it is to embrace a relaxed atmosphere. The true test of an advanced student is to embrace a harmonious balance of control, focus, strength, and relaxation. Always remember "softness is strength" and your inner calm will embrace much more strength and control than a show of muscle flexing, grunting, and expending all your energy.

Environment—As an advanced student, try an outdoor practice at least three times a month, weather permitting. When you practice outdoors, you soak up at least ten times the amount of *prana* energy and can actually feel the soothing touch of plants and trees. The ultimate experience for an advanced student is to practice outdoors in a mild climate with minimal clothing, and then takes a plunge into a clean river, ocean, or spring for dessert.

If the great outdoors is not an option, create an indoor paradise with lots of plants and a supply of fresh air. Wheat grass grown in flats is one of the most beneficial plants known to oxygenate the atmosphere. Many experiments have been conducted showing the benefits of growing wheat grass indoors for increased oxygen, pollution control, and enhanced *prana* energy. However, you cannot always control all these situations, especially if you are practicing in someone else's studio. As a advanced student, you should strive to find comfort in all situations and make the best of what you have.

Instruction Category—As an advanced student, pick one teacher as your base, yet study from many different teachers in the larger spectrum of things. No one teacher has all the answers, no matter what they tell you. Even if your teacher is highly recommended, famous, and of guru status, if they claim their system is the best ever and encourage you never to seek other instruction, then they have failed at their own yoga practice!

WHAT TO EXPECT

As an advanced student of Sadhana Yoga Flow, you should strive to incorporate all aspects of this system; yoga, cross-training with other exercise, diet, and enhanced state of mind. If you can gradually embrace the full spectrum, there is almost nothing you cannot accomplish. You will be rewarded with ultimate physical and mental health, as your inward harmony reflects into whatever life has in store for you.

Remember above all else to enjoy the journey, look forward to your practice, and remember that the object is not to achieve the most advanced posture, even if you are practicing at this level. As an advanced student, it is a good idea to strive toward connecting all of your postures together with *vinyasas* and rest in between your postures less, only when you feel it is necessary. Strive toward having a continuous flow of practice. Feel the energy flow between your yoga postures and let your practice look like a soft poetic dance, yet embrace power, confidence, and strength.

Moving Forward

As an advanced student, it is good to periodically go back and practice some routines from the intermediate and advanced-level workout. This will give you the opportunity to concentrate on developing a nice flow with a less demanding yoga workout. Then you can carry these concepts of flow with some newfound self-confidence into your advanced level practice.

As an advanced student, there will be other times when it will be to your overall advantage not to practice advanced yoga for several days, or even refrain from the physical aspects of yoga practice altogether for a whole week. I know this sounds counterproductive, yet advanced yoga practice is a very powerful energy exchange and you periodically need to take a complete rest. During this time you can do other physical activities, or just rest and relax

Yoga Postures and Vinyasas

As an advanced student, you should try to practice more difficult routines on a regular basis and hold postures longer. You can practice four or five times each week, with a session of length of anywhere from 60 minutes to 2 hours each practice. In time you can practice up to six days a week, with extended practice lengths. Some days you may find your personal practices are as long as 2½ hours and other days only 60 minutes. Don't be obsessed with how much time you spend; be mentally flexible, listen to your body, and do what is best for you.

Achieving All Postures

Postures which are very difficult for you, even after years of practice, could mean your body type is not best suited for this posture. If you have a good understanding of a yoga posture, you can still teach it, even if you cannot yet achieve this posture yourself. Although always remember the object of yoga is not to see who has the most flexibility and strength, but to get in touch with the natural flow of *prana*.

HARD AND SOFT FLOW YOGA

I have suggested a *vinyasa* for each yoga posture, yet you can choose to work harder, or choose to take it easy. Even as an advanced student, you need to read the instructions for each individual yoga posture, focus on the energy plane of practice, and control your level of workout. Remember to structure your practice with a balance of both ends of the spectrum. In the long run softness is power and when it blends with strength it creates a wonderful melody.

YOGA SEQUENCING

Yoga sequencing is designed to enhance your whole body physically and mentally. It is important for you to follow the proper order of yoga postures as laid out in the routines I have provided. If you randomly pick any yoga posture and disregard the proper sequencing, you will have a much larger risk of injury, loose a great deal of the energy flow, and become tired and unfocused after the practice.

INSTRUCTIONS FOR THE ROUTINES

The two workout routines listed in this chapter are presented as either short or long, depending on how much time you have to practice. The times each routine will take are only general guidelines: remember that you should never rush your routine; yoga is best when you take your time.

If you choose the long routine and then find out you do not have enough time to finish, start where you left off the next time. However, always start your routine with breathing and yoga warm-ups, then add the postures, and finish with cool-down exercises, more breathing, and deep relaxation. If you only get halfway through your routine, then save time to do your deep relaxation and at the next practice start with breathing, warm-ups, and then take up where you left off.

SITTING AND BREATHING

As an advanced student, challenge yourself now and then by holding your seated postures a bit longer. Listen to your body, and if you have pain in the joints avoid Lotus Posture until you recover.

Yoga Warm-up Exercises

Even at the advanced level, warm-ups are still a very important aspect of your practice. Always take time to warm up and try to be kind to your body. Warm-up exercises are an important step to fulfilling your enhanced endurance and aerobic qualities within yoga practice, so don't skip these wonderful exercises in order to save time.

Sun Salutation Information

In this level routine you will notice I have added two separate Sun Salutations. You can alternate between the two at separate practice sessions, or practice a minimum of two repetitions of each. All the Sun Salutations in this program are very beneficial for advanced-level students, and you should try to incorporate the variety into your ongoing practice.

STANDING POSTURES

The standing postures in the advanced-level routines connect with *vinyasas* for a great way to get in touch with your flowing *prana* energy. Once every few weeks you should close your eyes during your standing postures in order to enhance balance and get in touch with the Earth's energy.

INVERSIONS AND COUNTER-STRETCHES

As an advanced student, you should be familiar with where your body is as you practice inversions. Several times a week strive to hold your inversions for twice the number of breaths. Create more self-confidence and stability by keeping in touch with the energy flow from the time you leave an upright posture, moving into your inversion, and back to an upright position.

There are, however, some circumstances when you should check with your doctor before attempting these postures. Inverted postures should be avoided if you have any of the following physical conditions:

- *a floating retina*
- *during your menstrual cycle*
- *severe injury to your neck*
- *glaucoma*
- *extreme high blood pressure*

LEG STRETCHES

As a advanced student, you should start to move deeper into your leg stretches, and once a week hold them for twice the breath count. Also, listen to your body and respect your limits. If you should pull or strain a muscle in practice, by all means back off, give it a rest, and try to cross-train with other physical activities.

BACK BENDS

As an advanced student, I suggest you rotate your back-bending postures between the full spectrum available. Cross-training with back stretches will allow you to practice a wider variety of postures and embrace a more holistic energy flow. Inhale as you enter your back bends and exhale as you exit. Be patient and breathe. When practicing Spinal Twist, remember to inhale as you enter the posture, exhale as you exit.

ARM BALANCE POSTURES

The arm balance postures can be quite challenging, even at the advanced level of practice. Within these arm balances you will receive muscle resistance training from lifting your own body weight. Breathe slowly and deeply, draw strength from the Earth, and keep your mind calm and relaxed. Remember to project the concept of "softness is strength." An advanced student should refine this and become one with the posture.

ADVANCED SHORT ROUTINE: (50–60 MINUTES)

SITTING AND BREATHING

Practice one of the following seated postures best suited for your present condition, and sit quietly, with good posture, for fifteen complete breaths. Let your breathing become smooth and fine, as you strive to expand your lungs with slow, deep inhalations and exhalations. As an advanced student, you should try to feel the energy moving through your body and be attentive to embracing a spiritual element. For variety and a well-balanced practice, choose a different posture each time you practice.

Advanced students should be attentive to a smooth entrance and exit with these inversions.

Shoulder Stand	(see pg. 81)
Fish or Bridge (Counter-Stretch)	(see pg. 84 or 85)

LEG STRETCHES

As an advanced student, you can move deeper into your stretch as you feel the lines of energy opening. Remember to breathe as you are stretching, exhale, release stress and tension as you move slightly deeper into your stretch, inhale, embracing energy as you back off from the stretch slightly.

Staff Posture	(see pg. 87)
Expanded Seated Angle	(see pg. 93)

BACK BENDS

Cobra	(see pg. 100)
Upside-Down Bow	(see pg. 107)

SPINAL TWIST

Noose Posture	(see pg. 111)

ARM BALANCE

Advanced students can choose from a variety of arm balance postures available, the hardest being the Handstand.

Peacock	(see pg. 114)
Or	
Handstand	(See Page 120)

Corpse Posture—Deep relaxation (10–20 minutes)	(see pg. 140)

ADVANCED LONG ROUTINE
(1:30 HOUR TO 2 HOUR PRACTICE)

In order to retain the full potential of energy flow, follow this routine from start to finish in the order laid out. Once a month, go back and hold postures for twice the suggested amount of time, in each given routine. If you find you do not have enough time to complete this routine in your allotted amount of time, simply take relaxation and finish the last half of your practice the next session. An advanced student should be able to connect every posture together with suggested *vinyasas* from the posture instructions in Chapter 4.

SITTING AND BREATHING—

Perfect Posture or Lotus	(See Page 53)
Yoga Breathing (15 breaths)	(See Page 37)

YOGA WARM-UP EXERCISES

Please follow the order as laid out in this routine below; the postures are listed in order of sequence. Advanced students can cross-train with all other warm-ups.

Neck rolls and Shoulder rolls	(See Page 58, 59)
Cat Stretch (two repetitions)	(See Page 64)
Soft Touch *Vinyasa* I (upward)	(see pg. 143)
(on an alternate practice session)	
Muscle Power *Vinyasa* 3 (upward)	(see pg. 148)
Willow Tree	(See Page 63)
Sun Salutation—Soothing Touch (four repetitions)	(See Page 66)
Sun Salutation—Ultimate Power (four repetitions)	(See Page 71)

In the standing postures strive to move with your breath and visualize where you are and where you want to go.

Extended Triangle Posture	(See Page 123)
Twisted Extended Triangle Posture	(See Page 125)
Extended Side Angle Posture	(See Page 126)
Twisted Extended Side Angle Posture	(See Page 128)
Expanded Foot Posture (all variations)	(See Page 130)
Warrior I	(See Page 135)
Warrior II	(See Page 136)
Warrior III	(See Page 137)
Soft Touch *Vinyasa* I (downward)	(see pg. 143)
(on an alternate practice session)	
Muscle Power *Vinyasa* 3 (downward)	(see pg. 148)

INVERSIONS AND COUNTER-STRETCHES

Complete all of the postures in this section in the order they appear.

Headstand and variations	(See Page 76)
Child's Posture	(See Page 77)
Shoulder Stand	(See Page 81)
Plough	(See Page 83)
Fish	(See Page 85)
Bridge	(See Page 84)

Complete all of the postures in this section in the order they appear.

Staff	(see pg. 87)
Seated Forward Bend	(See Page 88)
Incline Plane	(See Page 90)
Head Knee Posture	(See Page 91)
Expanded Seated Angle	(See Page 93)
Expanded Foot Posture Variation 5	(See Page 133)
Shooting the Bow	(See Page 97)
Leg Behind Head	(See Page 98)
Boat Posture	(See Page 99)

BACK BEND POSTURES

Complete all of the postures in this section in the order they appear.

Cobra (3 repetitions)	(See Page 100)
Full Locust	(See Page 103)
Bow	(See Page 104)
Camel	(See Page 105)
Upside-Down Bow	(See Page 107)

SPINAL TWISTING POSTURES

Twist Posture I	(See Page 109)
Noose Posture	(See Page 111)

Complete all of the postures in this section in the order they appear.

Peacock	(See Page 114)
Scale	(See Page 116)
Scorpion	(See Page 117)
Crane	(See Page 118)
Sideways Crane	(See Page 119)
Handstand	(See Page 120)

BREATHING AND PRANAYAMA

Bellows Breathing	(See Page 40)
Lion Breathing Exercise (3 repetitions)	(See Page 42)
Alternate Breathing (2 repetitions)	(See Page 41)
Stomach Roll	(See Page 139)
Eye exercises	(See Page 139)

DEEP RELAXATION (10–20 MINUTES)

| Corpse Posture (Deep relaxation) | (See Page 140) |

PART III

———

CREATING HARMONY WITHIN FOR HEALTH AND LONGEVITY

RELAXING FOR
REJUVENATION

Stunning sunset paints the sky

'Tis warm beauty's embrace

Graceful birds soar the horizon

Whispers time, slow the pace

Now that you have an understanding of the physical requirements of Sadhana Yoga, I can begin to explain how to acquire that magical yogic attitude, or focused state of mind. The energy and grace harnessed within the yoga routine has unlimited positive effects as it soothes the body and mind. Now all you have to do is learn to unleash this powerhouse of potential *prana* and do some great things throughout you daily life.

The holistic approach of Sadhana Yoga reaches into every aspect of life, and is based on the importance of adopting healthier habits both physically and mentally. Whether your goal is to make small changes by taking a broad approach or instead to focus deeply on one aspect at a time, adopting any of the following elements can surely bring you closer to the pure flow of vital life force energy.

In our society we are all trained from a very young age to hurry through life. We are taught that losers finish last, and that time is money. This approach to life causes us all to encounter huge amounts of stress, tension, and lack of focus.

In Sadhana Yoga, winners finish last! The one who takes the time to ensure a full spectrum of relaxation will always achieve much more than those among us who are stressed out and are racing through every moment in life, without really knowing where they are going. Each and every moment in life is a very precious gift, and we should learn to taste the moment before you swallow the year. Many of the greatest things in life are contained within simplicity: you simply need to slow down in order to find them.

The Benefits of Relaxation

The benefits of relaxation are endless; unfortunately in today's fast-paced society few really get to experience the full spectrum of relaxation. If you are one of the few, then you are very fortunate. There is a popular misconception that relaxing means you are being lazy. In fact, just the opposite is true: when you take the time to embrace a full spectrum of quality relaxation, you will be much more productive, efficient, and focused with everything else you choose to accomplish.

Relaxation releases tension, stress, and fatigue from every part of your body as it soothes and quiets your mind, leaving you feeling tranquil and calm, yet still very alert and ready to respond to the world around you. The process of giving your body and mind proper relaxation is the best way to deal with your stress and tension, so that you react more calmly to the highs and lows of daily life.

Relaxation helps you deal with stress and enhances your overall energy reserves. A regular practice of relaxation has a great role to play in how you react to situations in daily life. For example, when something happens that usually drives you crazy—like losing your keys—your normal response might be to quickly build up inner turmoil and stress as you run frantically around searching for the lost item. After you've been practicing Sadhana Yoga for a few months, your response is likely to be much more rational and functional, as you stop, take a deep breath, clear your mind, and go about pursuing a solution in a controlled and efficient, yet relaxed manor.

When you're relaxed, you also tend to be more self-confident and have a more positive outlook. Many of us spend a lot of time thinking about things that we've done wrong in the past or could have done better, or worrying about things that we might have to deal with in the future. This train of thought creates a lack of self-confidence. Feeding your body and mind with proper relaxation encourages you to discard those self-defeating thoughts and to learn how to feel good about yourself.

Relaxation also helps to heal your body. Stress and tension often weakens your body's internal systems and makes you more susceptible to illness, injury, and even disease. In fact, stress is closely linked to heart disease, which is one of the major causes of death in our society. By helping you to relieve tension and stress, you can think of relaxation as one of the best medicines for your body.

Feeling the Stress

Tension and stress are a common reality for almost everyone. For example, you might feel stressed if you have to deal with financial matters, relationship problems, work in a competitive environment, or have to deal with multitasking and huge responsibilities. Stress can also occur within other areas of your personal life when you are dealing with injuries, sickness, or the pressure to exercise and stay healthy. There is also the constant stress of managing your life within a world filled with air pollution, water pollution, excessive noise, and toxins in our food.

The Good News

There are many ways to relieve stress. Within the Sadhana Yoga program I will show you many ways to release your stress, handle problems, soothe your brain, and focus better on finding solutions which will truly affect your whole life in a positive way. The first tool is what I call "The Less Stress List." See how many of the following techniques you can adapt to your life:

The Less Stress List:

1. Partake of some type of physical exercise, like yoga.

2. Hang out with friends when you need extra support, and have a good time: laughter is still the best medicine.

3. Take some time out of your day to breathe, relax, and unwind.

4. Turn your attention to the things you can control, and accept the things you cannot.

5. Strive to solve problems, not cover symptoms. Confront your stress and find solutions to work it out.

6. Become a neutral vessel: hear, see and take action without losing your emotional balance.

7. Eat a healthy diet and stay away from junk food.

Enjoying Leisure Activities

Leisure relaxation encompasses all aspects of sports and recreation, including enjoying hobbies, playing in nature, or chilling out. In all of these activities you can embrace many of your yoga techniques to assist you toward a higher quality of relaxation, instead of focusing on winning. With sports you can strive to do the best you can and make an effort to have a great time, whether you win or lose.

Sports and Recreation

Your leisure activities will assist you in your overall yoga practice, and your overall yoga practice will in turn assist you in your leisure relaxation. The idea that by practicing yoga, all other activities become counterproductive, nonspiritual, or nonbecoming to a yoga practitioner is a total misconception. Your training in yoga will assist you in excelling in many sports and games, by helping you achieve a clear focused mind and a strong and flexible body.

Many years ago I was an aspiring competitive surfer, living in Texas. The waves were terrible—you could find better waves in your bathtub—yet I dreamed of becoming a professional surfer. I knew that I was good at surfing, but not great. One year I saved all my money and with some help from my parents took a trip to Hawaii, where I discovered what real waves looked like. My ability at surfing the small, slow-moving waves in Texas was no match for the fast, very large, beautiful waves in Hawaii. After my visit to Hawaii, I returned to Texas, and shortly thereafter I was blessed to have yoga cross my path. Surfing in itself can be a very relaxing way to release stress and tension, yet with the magical touch of yoga, the feeling was totally wonderful.

As I practiced more yoga, something very magical started to happen with my surfing. My balance and flexibility improved, plus I felt an instant connection to the energy of the waves. With more yoga came endless self-confidence. Yoga had given me a soothing touch of energy, which was reflected in my movements on the waves. Through yoga I found a very intimate connection with the energy of the ocean: my surfing became a free flow of creative expression in sync with the energy of the waves. Needless to say my surfing ability went from being okay to extremely awesome and then off the charts. I was the first person from Texas to have been invited to compete in the world surfing championships.

I encourage you to add sports to your life. The aerobic and endurance factor of most sports will add a higher quality in your hard and soft form yoga practice. If possible try to practice a bit of yoga after sports or other physical activity: this can take tension out of your muscles, relax your mind, place your body back into proper alignment, and leave you feeling rejuvenated.

When practicing sports, try to use your yoga breathing to assist you in better focus and strength. Find your center just as you would focus in your yoga practice and put your flexibility to work to your advantage. Be in control and aware of your body at all times: this will help you to avoid injuries and create a stronger more focused manor of play. Remember to listen to your body and know your limits: if you are good at yoga, it does not mean you can run out and do a marathon in record time.

Hobbies

Hobbies encompass both physical and nonphysical activities. The yoga tradition suggests that what is important is maintaining a balance of activities. Physical hobbies will assist you in mental hobbies and mental hobbies will assist you in physical hobbies. Yoga will definitely assist you with your personal hobbies by making you more creative, self-confident, and focused. In turn your hobbies will serve as a balance from an overdose of yoga! A pleasant relaxing hobby is a great way to release tension and stress in your leisure time. Hobbies can also act as a creative outlet or expression of your ideas and talents.

Nature's Touch

Try to spend time in nature on a regular basis. Play, exercise, read, or do yoga in nature, and you will discover the feeling of a soothing touch, strength, and total relaxation all in one package. Of course, in the wrong conditions you might not find nature so soothing.

If you live in extreme weather conditions, try to find ways to have at least some of nature in your life. The ultimate experience is to practice your yoga outdoors near a waterfall, in the desert at sunset, among a meadow of flowers, on a mountaintop, or on a tropical beach.

The more time you spend in nature the better you will understand your yoga practice. However, there are some things to be cautious of when spending time outdoors. It is always important to dress properly for the weather and to minimize sun exposure. If you are exercising outdoors and are not properly dressed, it can be an unpleasant experience. If you are fair skinned and exercise in the middle of the day when the sun is the strongest, you will end up with a bad sunburn that will damage and be destructive to your skin in the long run. You can practice yoga or exercise on a very hot day if you stay in the shade and drink plenty of water. Yoga under the shade of a large tree on a very hot day is a wonderful experience. On the other end of the spectrum, if it is very cold outside, dress warmly; wear a hat and exercise in the sun.

Chilling Out

Sometimes it's wonderful to create some time for no particular purpose. Yoga can help you to manage your time and be more productive with your life, so that when you do have some downtime you can enjoy it fully. Every now and then it is good to just do nothing and find sanctuary in the quietness of the moment. Indoors or outdoors, enjoying your moments of downtime can be a very rejuvenating experience.

LETTING GO WITH YOGA DEEP RELAXATION

Yoga Deep Relaxation is without a doubt the most effective way to release stress and create a new outlook on life. Deep Relaxation has been an important part of yoga workout routines since the dawn of yoga practice. The yoga *asanas* systematically work every aspect of your physical body. In turn, you also need to rejuvenate and replenish your energies after your practice is finished.

Discovering Yoga Deep Relaxation

Yoga Deep Relaxation is different from simply relaxing in several ways. Yoga Deep Relaxation is a complete body recharge from head to toe: think of it as a concentrated version of all the best things about relaxing practiced in a relatively short amount of time. In this practice you are using focused yoga breathing techniques combined with the power of positive suggestion while you tense and relax each and every part of your body to achieve a soothing, peaceful, and rested euphoric feeling. Yoga Deep Relaxation is the most efficient way to create more energy, focus the mind, and enhance your organizational skills.

Steps to a Successful Yoga Deep Relaxation

The first step to beginning Yoga Deep Relaxation is to choose the right environment. Make sure you are comfortable, warm, and in a quiet setting. It is best to do this exercise on the firmness of the floor, using a yoga mat or blanket: lying on your soft bed might be too relaxing, as you are not looking to fall asleeep. Wear loose, comfortable clothing, yet make sure you are not too hot or too cold. In addition, you might want to use an eye pillow; this is a small beanbag-type cushion that will shield your eyes from light.

YOGA DEEP RELAXATION

BENEFITS

In this exercise you will release stress and tension from every area of your body and mind. You will lower your blood pressure, soothe your heart, and focus your mind. This is one of the most important aspects of your regular yoga practice, and you should always end every practice session with a complete deep relaxation. Failure to do so will result in a loss of energy, and a less effect yoga practice. This technique can also be used in your daily life to maintain you inner peace.

POSTURE PREPARATION

Yoga Deep Relaxation is best practiced when you are lying on you back in the *Savasana* Posture, which is also known as the Sponge or Corpse Posture (see Chapter 4 for complete instructions on this pose). In this position you are lying on the floor resembling the stillness of a corpse, yet soaking up the energy from the universe, much like a sponge soaks up water. Place a yoga mat or blanket on the floor and assume your posture. Some students find it useful to place an additional small pillow under their knees. Allow 10 to 20 minutes to complete the Yoga Deep Relaxation cycle.

1. Start from Corpse Posture, lying flat on your back, feet about one foot apart, with arms by your sides and palms facing upward. Once you are comfortable, you can begin to practice your Yoga breathing techniques. Maintain a slow, even rhythm as you completely fill your lungs on inhalations and completely empty your lungs on exhalations. As you practice slow deep breathing, think about relaxation each time you exhale. Strive to maintain your slow soft yoga breathing throughout the whole relaxation exercise.

2. Begin to tense and relax your muscles. Starting with your right leg, lift it off the floor about 12 inches, and tense every muscle in your whole leg for a few seconds, then slowly relax. Gently lower your right leg back to the floor on an exhalation.

3. Slowly lift your left leg up about 12 inches from the floor, tense every muscle in your whole leg for a few seconds, then slowly relax. Gently lower your left leg back to the floor on an exhalation.

4. Begin to tighten the muscles in your hips and buttucks for a few seconds, then relax and allow your gluteus muscles to melt into the floor on an exhalation.

5. Arch your back up off the floor, pressing down with your elbows and shoulders as you expand your chest up toward the sky. Hold for a few seconds, then slowly relax, lowering your back to the floor on an exhalation.

6. Give your back a counter-stretch by pressing your lower back into the floor. This is done by tightening your gluteus and stomach muscles as you press the lower back against the floor. Hold for a few seconds and relax completely on an exhalation.

7. Slowly lift your right arm about 12 inches from the floor, tensing all of its muscles. Hold this for a few seconds, then relax on an exhalation and lower your arm back to the floor.

8. Slowly lift your left arm about 12 inches from the floor, tensing all of its muscles. Hold this for a few seconds, then relax on an exhalation and lower your arm back to the floor.

9. Leaving your head on the floor, slowly roll your head to the right side, then slowly to the left side; now return your head to the center, exhale, and relax.

10. On your next inhalation, fill your mouth up with air, blowing your cheeks out like big balloons; hold for just a second or two, then relax and release the air.

11. Gently stretch all your facial muscles, then slowly relax them on an exhalation.

12. Close your eyes and take five very slow, deep inhalations and exhalations, clearing your mind.

13. Now you will begin your visual relaxation. You will visualize each part of your body and "tell" each muscle to relax. Starting with your feet, visualize a very relaxed feeling coming into your toes, relaxing the balls of your feet, releasing all the tension from the arches of your feet and your heels. Now release the tension from the tops of your feet and your ankles. Both of your feet will be completely and totally relaxed.

14. Visualize that relaxed feeling coming into your shins, relaxing your calf muscles. Now release all the tension from your knees, thighs, and hamstrings. With both of your legs completely relaxed from your waist all the way down to your toes, you allow your tensions to surrender to the Earth.

15. Now visualize that relaxed feeling moving into your gluteus muscles and slowly moving upward, as your lower back releases all the tension from your middle back and your upper back. Visually release all the tension from each vertebrae, starting with the back of your neck and moving slowly down all the way to the base of your spine. Allow all the tension to completely leave your back.

16. Feel the tension leaving your abdominal muscles, relaxing your ribs, releasing all the tension from your chest and your shoulders. This will leave your whole torso completely relaxed, from your shoulders to your waist.

17. Visually relax the backside of your neck, the sides of your neck, and underneath your chin. Allow your whole jaw to completely relax, releasing all those tensions from your lips, cheeks, and tongue.

18. Visually relax the area around your nose and your eyes, also releasing tension from your forehead and the sides of your face.

19. Take a slow soft inhalation and on your exhalation, visualize your heart and mentally ask your heart to relax. Take another slow soft inhalation and then

on your exhalation, visualize your brain, and mentally ask your brain to relax, calm your mind and release your negative thoughts. Clear your mind of all but the most pleasant and positive thoughts: perhaps you can visualize yourself in a beautiful place in nature, as you drift effortlessly in complete relaxation.

20. When you are finished, slowly stretch your arms up over your head on an inhalation, as you stretch your legs in the opposite direction, then relax and roll over to your right side, with arms and legs slightly bent. Remain here for a few breaths. Gradually come back to a sitting position and try to preserve the positive uplifting thoughts you created.

The more often you practice your deep relaxation, the better you will get at this wonderful technique. If you have trouble getting to sleep, try this deep relaxation exercise as a preface before you get into bed and you will find yourself sleeping soundly. The deep relaxation has also been used successfully in treating muscle spasms, anxiety, and for releasing chronic pain. To assist with relieving pain in specific areas of your body, simply follow the instructions for the above relaxation, then focus your attention on the area of your body where you are experiencing pain. Turn your attention to your area of focus, practicing slow deep breathing, then on exhalations, think about releasing the pain. The results are quite profound after only five minutes.

When to Practice Yoga Deep Relaxation

The best time to do your Yoga Deep Relaxation is right after your physical yoga *asana* practice. You may find this technique valuable at any time of day or night, so feel free to step out of your busy schedule whenever you feel as if you need to have a soothing break. If you are having a stressful day, take a few quiet moments to embrace this wonderful deep relaxation technique: although less effective, you can even practice this deep relaxation while you are seated at your desk!

SURRENDERING TO RESTFUL SLEEP

Sleep is a very important and necessary aspect in your Sadhana Yoga program. You may have heard stories of *yogis* going without sleep for long periods of time. This is not a good idea, because trying to go without sleep, or limiting your much-needed sleep, will only serve to weaken your immune system and distract you from your vital life force energy.

In today's world we are constantly pushing each other to go faster, to reduce sleep, and to work more. This will ultimately result in a weakened immune system, a general lack of energy, and a scattered, unfocused mind. Sleeping is an important part of relaxation. Try to get eight hours of sleep each night: in the long run you will be rewarded many times over.

But even when you are sleeping, there are different kinds of sleep. You can basically divide sleep into two categories, restful sleep and nonrestful sleep. Yes, it is possible to sleep and not get an adequate amount of rest. I am sure you have had many nights when your sleep is very broken, either by bad dreams or segmented sleep patterns, and you do not experience total surrender to a deep, restful sleep. After such a night you usually awake feeling very tired, unfocused, and a bit slow to respond. A restful sleep occurs when you lie down in bed, have some pleasant thoughts, and then drift into a very relaxing and undisturbed rest. Upon awaking you feel refreshed, energized, and ready to seize the day.

Helpful Yogic Hints for Good Sleep

When talking about getting a good night's sleep, there are several variables which can help contribute to your success. A good night's rest really shows on your overall performance. In order to achieve a good night's sleep, you need to improve many elements of your day, including your sleeping environment, your level of exercise and activity, and your diet. Taking all these things into consideration will greatly assist you in achieving consistently restful sleep.

ENVIRONMENT—The environment you sleep in has a great effect on your sleep success. Treat your bedroom as a sanctuary for sleeping. Choose a room which is quiet and comfortable, assuring ample darkness for you to rest, undisturbed. Create a comfortable environment by having plenty of fresh air in your room, extra blankets in the winter, and light, cool sheets in the summer. Make sure your room retains the proper temperature which makes you comfortable, even under heavy blankets. Another great suggestion is to have plants in your bedroom. Plants oxygenate the air and filter pollution, both of which will assist you in getting a restful sleep. The best plant for oxygenating the air is wheat grass. You can usually buy an inexpensive flat of wheat grass from your local health-food store. Transplant this wheat grass in an appealing flowerpot and place a pot on both sides of your bed.

PHYSICAL ACTIVITY BEFORE SLEEP—Work and play hard and you will be rewarded with a good night's sleep. However, if you do not get an adequate amount of exercise—especially aerobic exercise—then the chances of a good night's sleep are greatly lessened. Also, exercising immediately before going to bed can keep you up for hours until your body slows down enough to fall asleep. Moderate sustained exercise like yoga practice, coupled with yoga breathing, will assist you in achieving a good night's sleep.

Aside from physical exercise, try to simplify your home routine after supper. Do not watch television or surf the Internet right before you go to bed: these activities actually stimulate brain activity and can prevent you from getting restful sleep.

EATING BEFORE BEDTIME—Meals eaten throughout your day can have an impact on you sleep patterns, especially the foods you eat at the end of the day. Eating lots of sugary foods, spicy foods, garlic, chocolates, or coffee can keep you up all night. Eating juicy fruit or drinking alcohol, caffeinated teas, or carbonated beverages right before bed will often wake you up in the middle of the night when your bladder needs to be relieved.

On the other hand, if you eat a balanced diet with plenty of fresh, raw, unprocessed rich green salads, moderate fruits, vegetables, raw nuts and seeds, and eliminate processed junk food from your plate, you should find it much easier to get to sleep. Also, if possible, try to have your evening meal before 7 P.M., eating too late can also disrupt your sleep.

Additional Sleeps Aids

To further enhance your sleep, you might think about trying some of the following techniques:

DEEP RELAXATION AND BREATHING—One of the best things you can do for yourself is to practice Yoga Deep Relaxation and deep breathing techniques. The Yoga Deep Relaxation in combination with yoga breathing is one of the best techniques you can use to assist you in a restful night's sleep. Refer to the yoga relaxation exercise and practice it right before you go to sleep. The results are quite wonderful.

SOOTHING RESTFUL HERBS—Within the spectrum of herbs, there are plants which will energize you and others which can calm you down. Try drinking a cup of chamomile or peppermint tea at least one hour before you want to go to bed. Drinking warm tea is best; however, you can use an herbal tincture. Go to your local health store and you will find some tea combinations which are labeled for aid in sleeping. Another herbal sleeping aid is to relax before bedtime in a warm Epsom salts bath, with a little tea tree oil or wheat grass oil poured into the bathwater. Soak for up to twenty minutes to get the full effects.

LIGHT MASSAGE—The soothing touch of a light massage will take tension out of your muscles, relax your mind, and greatly assist you in getting good sleep. However, a deep tissue massage or a more aggressive massage may keep you up.

NATURE—If you have trouble getting to sleep, try taking a short to moderate walk outdoors. Walk slowly and enjoy the soothing touch of nature. Try camping out now and then, sleeping out under the stars and enjoying the essence of nature.

MUSIC—The last music you hear before going to sleep can also have an impact on your sleep. Listen to something which leaves you with a good feeling and in the mood to completely relax and drift to sleep. The soothing voice of another has long since been used to melt us into a restful sleep. Adults and children alike can both use a bedtime story now and then, to soothe our tired brains and warm our soul.

READING AND WRITING—For many years reading before bed has been very effective in creating restful quality sleep for me. As a student of yoga, you might try reading about philosophy and the background of yoga, or help your kids with a yoga coloring book. Writing is also a very relaxing way to assist you into a restful sleep. Write about pleasant things in life, try composing some poetry, or write a letter to a friend. Try to avoid working on the computer late at night, because the energy from the computer can keep you from getting to sleep. Revert back to the old ways and try handwriting a nice letter instead.

Improving Your Dream State

You can improve your dream state simply by leading yourself through the same type of yoga relaxation as listed earlier in this chapter, only enhancing it by telling a story instead of visualizing nature. You can interject a warm and soothing story which will in turn affect the quality of your dreams in a positive way. If you are concerned about your own peace of mind in sleep, you can record your own story and relaxation exercise, and play this recording as you go to bed. If you are a singer or a musician, try recording your own soothing music and play it before sleep.

MEDITATING

TO SOOTHE

YOUR SOUL

The quiet mind of a yogi
Seeks the power of the whole universe
The power of the whole universe
Seeks the tranquility of the quiet mind

Meditation is a multipurpose tool with many wonderful benefits. Meditation releases stress and tension, helps you become more organized, and at the same time assists you to create harmony within. The benefits of meditation affect your external life as well. Outwardly you will generate energy with a focused soothing touch, yet remain confident and strong.

You may associate meditation only with monks, nuns, sages, and yoga teachers, but the reality is that people of all walks of life are meditating, including the postal worker, the bank vice preisent, the sanitation worker, the dishwasher, the attorney, and of course, rock stars! Anyone and everyone who wants to improve the quality of his or her mind and life is trying meditation.

Many think of meditation as the absence of thought. However, nothing could be further from the truth. In meditation you are eliminating the clutter in your head as you discipline your mind. A merging of inward power into a very organized and focused resource. Meditation is the means by which you can calm your restless mind until it becomes still, then focus all your energy and attention on one thought or area. Meditation is therefore not the goal, but only a tool that helps you connect to the vital life force. Through meditation you are essentially training your mind to work in harmony with your body, allowing you to reach your full potential.

Seeking the Roots of Meditation

Meditation is an ancient art that is practiced by many cultures and religions. However, meditation in itself is not a religious or faith-based activity. Many world religions have used meditation techniques to enhance their existing faith. Think of meditation as a mental exercise to help get your mind in shape; what you choose to do with your rejuvenated thoughts are up to you.

For example, the Native American shamans, or healers, reached enlightened states through drumming, chanting, dancing, healthy diet, and meditation. These activities often led them into a higher state of mind which lasted for hours or even days. During this enhanced state of mind the shamans were in touch with the vital life force energy and found a greater connection with the power and softness of nature. During this meditative state they often had visions of plants, which helped them to seek medicinal plants for healing.

Meditation is also a popular technique among Buddhists and is said to have been used by Buddha himself. After Buddha had practiced a restrictive diet, simplicity of lifestyle, and different styles of yoga for many years, he felt he had looked everywhere for enlightenment, but to no avail. He realized that he had overlooked the inward path, so he began to practice meditation. Later, he spent seven days and nights observing his mind while in a constant meditative state. When he emerged from his meditative state, he understood the nature of our existence, and therefore was named "the awakened one," or *Buddha*.

In yoga practice, meditation is one of the eight limbs along the path to enlightenment. Practiced by itself, meditation is called *Raja* Yoga. In Sanskrit *raja* means "king," and *yoga* means "union or bring together," so *Raja Yoga* is the quest to become king of your mind, to focus, tune, relax, and control it while working in unison with your physical body.

The traditional term for meditation is *bhavana*, which translates as "mental and emotional development." Just as you can develop your body through physical exercise, you can also develop your mind through mental exercise. Once you have a more focused mental power, you can begin to work on strengthening your own emotional development. Experienced *yogis* and *yoginis* have more control over their emotions. This does not mean that showing your emotions is a bad thing, yet there are times when control can produce a positive reaction and become a grand asset to communication.

The Practice of Meditation

The meditation techniques that are commonly practiced today focus on the ability to control restless thoughts. By letting your mind flow and empty itself of distractions, then you can concentrate your power of thought into one area or concept.

THE POWER OF MEDITATION

With meditation, the saying "The journey is everything" fits very appropriately. After you gain control over your mind, you can guide your thoughts and strive to achieve some of the following:

1. The ability to choose not to dwell upon every thought which comes into your mind, but having the ability to throw away the ones of lesser value.

2. The knowledge that you can take your mind off negative emotions such as hate, worry, fear, and anxiety simply by choosing to think of something else.

3. The ability to organize your mind into catagories of thought, such as positive thoughts, negative thoughts, memories, fantasy, illusions, and reality.

4. The ability to enhance your memory and recall things of importance at will.

5. The ability to be able to put things into proper perspective, yet not allowing this to interfere with your emotional stability.

6. The ability to enhance your appreciation for life's simple gifts, such as the col-

ors of springtime flowers, the sound of a running creek, children playing, or the gentle touch of a loved one.

This inward focus leads you to the ability to contemplate your true essence, leading to *samadhi*, or self-realization, and the union with the universe. In Sadhana Yoga, the goal of your meditation can be divided up into two different categories. **Personal Meditations** are targeted at achieving stress reduction and higher mental and spiritual states of mind. **Specific Meditations** are targeted to create insight into specific ideas, or objects of focus. The first category is a necessary base in order to achieve the second.

MEDITATION VS. SLEEPING

The meditation and relaxation techniques used in Sadhana Yoga are similar to a state of sleep, yet you remain awake and very aware. This awareness is what makes meditation and relaxation so effective and powerful. When you sleep, you close your eyes and, with luck, drift off, passing through a dream phase along the way. In sleep you are not in control of your journey. Your mind is in a subconcious mode, and you cannot control where your thoughts choose to go. In meditation and relaxation you strive to gain conscious control over your mind and lead your thoughts into the area of your choice.

TOUCHING THE POWER OF STILLNESS

When you think of the meaning of power within the human form, you might envision a strong weight lifter with rippling muscles, or a world-class athlete whose body is capable of remarkable physical feats. These people truly have strength, and yet they are expending energy and depleting their reserves in their athletic practice. In meditation and relaxation, you create power without depleting your energy by remaining completely still. In fact, you are replenishing and rejuvenating the energy that you have depleted through other activities. This is why you should try to practice meditation at the end of your yoga session: you are trying to leave your exercise mat feeling better than when you first started your practice. Your energy is felt as both softness and strength as you tap into the vital life force, all the while remaining calm and relaxed.

PHYSICAL BENEFITS OF MEDITATION

You can use your meditation to release stress, gain strength, and mental focus, lower your blood pressure, enhance your self-confidence, and create inner peace. By calming your thoughts and focusing your mind, you can release all your stress and gain mental clarity. Medical studies have proven that if you can lower your levels of stress and tension, you can reduce blood pressure levels and lower the risk of heart attack, stroke, and other stress-related illnesses.

Other studies have shown benefits from meditation and the release of stress and tension as an avenue to enhance your immune system. Your mind is a very powerful tool, which can assist you in preventing and overcoming sickness. I am sure you have noticed that when you are mentally run-down you tend to get sick more easily, or have a harder time recovering. Meditation can also help to regulate the functions of your endoncrine system. Your endocrine system is responsible for secreting hormones into your boodstream, which then travel to the area of your body needed to exert their effect. Many studies have also proven meditation is effective in the treatment of migraine headaches, anxiety, depression, and hostility.

YOUR EMOTIONS AND MEDITATION

Meditation helps you to get grounded: to feel connected with life and all living things. Through meditation you will also be able to improve your communication skills. Communication starts from within: if you cannot "talk" with yourself, you will have a hard time communicating with others. Meditation can enhance your motor skills and increase the self-confidence necessary for better commmunication.

Meditation can also help to improve your ability to concentrate and allows for clearer thinking. You can become more creative and cultivate joy and happiness, love and compassion, and selfless action. You're better able to process your emotions, which can help develop healthier relationships with family, friends, and lovers.

Meditation helps you reach the ultimate bliss and connection with the universe. This connection is called *samadhi*, or "enlightenment." Enlightenment means different things to different people, but is generally characterized by feeling the complete peace of all life, understanding the nature of your existence, and seeing yourself as a part of the whole as you observe life without ego. I believe we all pass in and out of *samadhi* throughout our lives. Through the practice of meditation you stand a greater chance of visiting *samadhi* more often, or staying in this state of mind for long periods of time.

Beginning the Process

CREATING A SACRED SPACE WITHIN

During meditation, you are actually cultivating the sacred space that is your soul. This is a peaceful place only you can find when you quiet the clutter and confusion of your mind.

It is in this sacred place where you are free of stress and tension as the mind is calm, at peace, and clear. As time passes, you will be able to find your way to your own sacred place whenever you need it. If you are faced with a stressful situation, you can instantly locate this space to relax, unwind, and find sanctuary. Creating inner harmony is much like taking a much-needed vacation. Paradise comes from within, as Henry David Thoreau said: "You can travel the world over to find the beautiful, yet you must carry it with you, or you will find it not."

CREATING A SACRED SPACE AROUND YOU

The first step in preparing to meditate is to choose a location. This location will become a haven where you can go to find your inner sacred space. Take time to cultivate this sacred garden, as it will become your center for meditation and rejuvenation. Create your sacred space with plants, art, or ideas that make you more comfortable, at peace, and relaxed. Utilize this as your warm and cozy spot to practice yoga, relax, breathe, and meditate. Go to your sacred space anytime to touch your heart and find the ultimate best within you!

If you choose an indoor location, choose a private spot that has good air flow and offers few distractions. I have a little room with an altar in my house. An altar is just a name for a space, like a little table or a mantel, that holds objects and photos that remind people of their own spirituality and their connection to the Earth. My altar has special plants, a few candles, some rocks and precious stones I have collected from my journeys, and pictures that are dear to me. You can decorate your own altar space with anything that connects you to your own spiritual self. Then, of course, add some pleasant music and good lighting.

You can also choose to meditate outdoors. You don't have to go anywhere special, you can create a beautiful space right in your own yard. Maybe you can put a bench near some soothing bushes or trees and plant some flowers. Perhaps even add a fountain. Make this space a healing, nurturing place that you enjoy spending time in. Let this be your own personal sactuary, a place where you treat yourself well and allow the environment to help assist with a soothing touch.

MUSIC FOR MEDITATORS

Music can help assist you to still your restless mind and set the mood for your meditation practice. Ultimately you have the choice with which music is most effective in assisting you with meditation. See the Resources section for a list of music that is appropriate for meditation.

Whenever you enter your sacred space, make sure that you are comfortable. Believe it or not, your clothing during meditation plays an important factor. Try to wear something that is loose-fitting, made with natural fibers, and does not restrict your blood flow. Make sure you are comfortable without being too warm or too cold. Remember that when you stay still for a long period of time your extremities might get cold, so think about wearing socks or gloves if you experience these sensations, or have a light blanket handy.

Walking the Sacred Path to Meditation

In the practice of meditation there is a preliminary foundation you must first journey through in order to achieve quality meditation. Some of these same techniques are used in your yoga *asana* practice. Just as you must build a strong foundation before you put a roof on your house, you must first practice the foundations to meditation. These beginning stages include posture, breathing, relaxation, sense withdrawal, and concentration. Once they are complete, then you can move gracefully into a medititive state of mind.

YOGA POSTURES TO ENHANCE MEDITATION

Yoga practice can be one step on the path to meditation. Yoga *asanas* create balance and union within your total body health. If you practice yoga postures before you meditate you will be more relaxed, balanced, mentally focused, and find it easier to control your mind. Ideally practicing a balanced yoga routine before your meditation will greatly increase the overall benefits, especially for beginners, because many of the concepts of yoga exercise will complement your atmosphere for meditation. However, you can certainly meditate at a separate time from your *asana* yoga practice.

Before you begin your meditation exercise, you first need to choose a yoga posture you wish to meditate in. Try meditating in a few different postures and see what feels comfortable to you. Review Chapter 4 to learn more details on each posture.

Perfect Posture: Sit in a cross-legged position, with your knees bent and feet pulled in toward your torso, without placing your feet on opposite thighs. If your feet start to fall asleep, separate them so your legs don't push on your ankles. You may also place a pillow under your buttocks to assist in better posture. If your hips are very tight, you might place another pillow that supports under your knees as well.

Lotus Posture: For students with open hips and flexible knees. Sit on the floor, with your ankles folded on top of opposite thighs. Your hands are resting on extended knees, with palms facing upward and forming *Jnana Mudra* with your fingers. Strive to keep your spine straight and shoulders back. Be aware of your knees in full Lotus Posture, don't stay too long, or you can injure your knees. Listen to your body!

Half Lotus: This posture is just like the Lotus Posture only you place one leg on your opposite thigh instead of both. Your hands are resting on extended knees, with palms facing upward and forming *Jnana Mudra* with your fingers. Strive to keep your spine straight and shoulders back. You should also be aware of your knees in Half Lotus Posture; don't stay too long, or you can injure your knees. It is also a good idea to switch legs the next time you sit, in order to achieve a balance in flexibility.

Thunderbolt: The Thunderbolt is a kneeling posture. Sit on your heels, with your knees folded up underneath you. You can sit on a small pillow between your legs, which will also help to correct bad posture. Fold your hands onto your lap, with your palms facing upward, one on top of the other.

Sitting in a Chair: If these yoga postures are not comfortable for you, or if you are practicing meditation during a work break, try sitting upright in a chair with feet firmly on the floor, supporting your own back, with a firm pillow if necessary. Place your feet and legs about a foot apart and parallel. Your hands should be resting in your lap or on your thighs.

YOGA BREATHING TECHNIQUES FOR MEDITATION

In the Sadhana Yoga program I have refined yoga breathing even further to enhance your meditation. The type of breathing used in yoga is called *ujjayi*, which translates as meaning "victorious breath." It is quite different from regular breathing, but it isn't really complicated at all. You can think of yoga breathing as having three distinct qualities:

The complete breath: With each breath, completely fill your lungs with air on an inhalation, called *puraka*, and completely empty your lungs on an exhalation, called *rechaka*. The exhalation is just as important as your inhalation: make a conscious effort to exhale completely.

Slow deep breathing: In Sadhana Yoga your breathing is slow, steady, deep, and rhythmic, which creates a calm and relaxed mind; it also enables you to take more oxygen into your lungs, leaving you feeling refreshed and invigorated after practice. We are living in a fast-paced world; allow your breathing to be an exception to this rule. Many yoga students try to rush the breath and in the long run sacrifice much energy and relaxation concepts.

Sound breathing (*ujjayi*): Yoga breathing involves the technique of inhaling and exhaling air through your nose. As you breathe in, tighten your throat muscles allowing the incoming air to make a soft, hissing sound on the back of your throat. This enables you to control the rate of time for your inhalation and exhalation. This tranquil, meditative sound in combination with your slow, deep, and calculated breathing pattern contributes to enhancing your overall energy, calming of your body and mind, enabling you to center your thoughts on your practice. In meditation practice you will use very light *ujjayi* breathing, which menas you will allow the sound to be very subtle, compared to your yoga posture practice, where you will allow the sound breathing to be very powerful, feeling the air pass over your throat, and finally passing out of your nose.

MINDFULNESS BREATHING

Most meditation techniques begin by focusing on the act of breathing. Focusing on your breathing will clear your mind as a preparation for meditation practice. A very useful technique for beginners is to count breaths. You may want to try counting after each exhalation. For example, take in a breath, push out a breath and count one; continue to a count of ten.

The second stage of mediation breathing is to calmly observe your breath and the sensations involved with breathing as you notice the air passing through your nose and into your lungs, being warmed by your body, and then moving calmly back out. You should start your yoga breathing as soon as you begin your meditation practice and continue with the slow, deep, fluid, rhythmic breathing until your practice is over. Continue with your controlled breathing as you calm and relax your mind with each inhalation and exhalation, feel and hear the air enter your nose and swirl past your throat.

Embracing Relaxation

Relaxation is an essential step along the path toward meditation. When you are relaxed, you tend to be more self-confident and hold a positive outlook on life. Many of us spend time thinking about things that we've done wrong or could have done better, or worrying about things that we might have to deal with in the future. This train of thought creates negative reactions and a lack of self-confidence, and just plain allows you to beat yourself up. Feeding your body and mind with proper relaxation encourages you to discard those self-defeating thoughts and feel good about yourself. It teaches you to be here now and live in the moment!

You cannot jump into meditation practice without first establishing a good relaxation environment within your body and mind. Many of the concepts of relaxation are interlaced with the concepts of meditation, such as posture, breath, and mental attitude. For complete instructions on how to relax, review Chapter 8.

By practicing a balanced yoga routine with deep breathing, you will have a much greater ability to maintain relaxation on a regular basis. Before meditation, you should either practice a balanced yoga routine or take a few moments to completely relax before your meditation. Here is a basic relaxation exercise to use as a foundation to help you get started on your path of meditation.

Pre-Meditation Relaxation Exercise

1. Choose a seated yoga position, or sit in a supportive chair. Maintain good posture with your spine straight and shoulders back. Fold your hands in your lap, or extend your hands out over your knees in *Jnana Mudra*.

2. Clear your thoughts and make yourself comfortable, as you bring your awareness to your breathing. Consciously practice slow deep breathing, completely filling your lungs on inhalations, and completely emptying your lungs in exhalations. Be aware of the sensation of breath and think relaxing thoughts on exhalations, as you slowly lengthen your inhalations and exhalations.

3. Release all negative thoughts, empty your mind from school, work, relationships, personal problems, or world affairs. Practice being in the moment by creating a passive mind and concentrate on something very pleasant. Congratulations, you have now laid a solid foundation and are on your way to a successful meditation.

SENSE WITHDRAWAL

The next stage along the path to meditation is what *yogis* call sense withdrawal. This is the fifth limb of the eight-limbed path to enlightenment. Many of its concepts are contained within your relaxation foundation: as you move into relaxation, you are actually embracing sense withdrawal as a means to relax. In this practice you are overriding outside distractions and turning your focus inward. You ignore outside sounds and release wandering thoughts. Observe your posture and listen to your breathing, as you become one with your inward journey.

Sense Withdrawal Exercises:

1. **Attention Without Attachment**—If you are successful at sense withdrawal, noises and other outside distractions will not disturb your meditation. You will

be able to recognize and be aware of outside movements and noises, yet they will not let your emotions and thoughts veer off course. This technique is called Attention Without Attachment, to be aware of all things, yet focused on your train of thought. Ignore outward sounds, release wandering thoughts, and focus your attention onto your posture. Become aware of your spinal alignment and strive to sit up straight, make a conscious effort to keep your shoulders open, and expand your chest.

2. **Focus on Breath**—Be aware of every aspect of your breathing. Feel the air as it enters and exits your nose. Visualize your lungs expanding on your inhalations and contracting on your exhalations. Think relaxing thoughts every time you exhale.

3. **Relax Muscle Tension**—In your mind, visit each area of your body, mentally suggesting to each of your muscles to completely relax. Listen to your heart beating and visualize your heart distributing oxygenated blood to all areas of your body.

CONCENTRATION

Now that you have embraced sense withdrawal, you have moved a bit further along the path toward a meditative state of mind. The next step is concentration. In the yogic tradition concentration is the sixth limb on the eight-limbed path of enlightenment. Concentration is the method used to narrow your quality of thought onto one particular point of interest. During concentration you are focusing your attention on a particular object, idea, subject, or thought. Your thoughts are relaxed yet you still have to make an effort to stay in this state of mind. In concentration you move a bit futher toward meditation, where your thoughts become effortless within a more relaxed state of mind. In meditation you no longer have to think about focusing your thoughts; you become one with the natural flow of energy.

In order to begin your concentration you first have to choose an object, idea, or problem to concentrate upon. Your area of focus has a direct influence on your area of meditation. In concentration and meditation you will have basically two choices:

Personal Concentration is geared to help you relax, release your stress, and ultimately create higher mental and spiritual states of mind. For this area you would fix your concentration onto internal avenues of amplified relaxation, self-confidence, personal health, nature visualizations, contemplation of the universe, or the spiritual avenues of your choice.

Specific Concentration is geared toward a single object, idea, thought, or problem. In this area you would first choose your subject and then allow your attention to move into this one specific area. Perhaps it is a canoe you are building, techniques of dance, ways to better organize your garage, a means to solve a personal problem, or even something as complex as how you would solve world affairs.

Concentration Exercise

I. Begin concentration by completing the stages of relaxation and sense withdrawal. Once you have completed these stages, pick your area of concentration from the above catagories and fix your attention on this area.

2. **Observation Around Subject**—Now that you have an area to concentrate on, you need to expand your focus to the widest area around your topic. This is a means by which you can explore anything and everything which has a connection to your subject. If your mind wanders off course, just remind yourself of the main focus and gently bring your attention back. For example, if your focus was on organizing your garage, you might first explore the benefits of the project: when is the best time to start this job, who will help you with this, where will you take the throwaway items, and what will you wear.

3. **Concentrating Your Focus**—Now that you have explored the peripheral reaches of your subject, it is time to tighten the field of thought until you have a very close, defined area of focus right around your topic. If this area is your garage organization, you would now focus more on the specific items in your garage, where you want to place these items, and which ones you need to throw away.

FINDING YOUR MEDITATION STYLE

Now that you have successfully completed your concentration exercise, you may move into your meditation. All you have to do is decide which style of meditation you are going to practice. When you first start meditating, your thoughts will be restless and scattered, and you may try a few techniques until you find the one that really works for you. I have listed several different meditation techniques you can try. Always remember that this is your own personal journey and you will do best to find which method works best for you. Take a seated pose, and give meditation a try:

SOUND MEDITATION

Repeating a meaningful word or saying. Many people like to meditate using a mantra, which is the repetition of a single word or phrase. Some use the word OM (pronounced "aum"). This word is significant as it translates as symbolizing our connection to the infinite universe. You may want to create a mantra that is meaningful to you. Try something simple, such as "Health Is Wealth," or "Kindness Speaks Through Its Actions." Some students like to concentrate on ideas they want to manifest in their own personal lives (perhaps something like "Strength through Softness").

    Chanting. Many religions use chanting or singing as a means of clearing the mind and connecting to the power of the universe. If you don't know any traditional chants about gods, saints, or sages, you can make up your own. Try listening to one of the recorded chantings I've listed previously, or even find some relaxing music which has a similar effect. You'll know when you've chosen the right music when you hear something that instantly makes you happy: try meditating on this.

    Soothing Music. You can choose light background music and meditate on the vibration, sound, and melody. For newcomers to meditation this is often an easy way to get started, as long as the music does not distract from the meditation.

VISUAL MEDITATION

Gazing at a photograph, drawing, inspirational image, or nature scene. Gazing at an image is a nice meditation technique. Color, depth of field, and meaning are all important aspects in choosing an image. For example, viewing photographs of nature or a personally signficant work of art can set a tone for successful meditation. If you are lucky enough to be able to meditate outside, you can gaze at a soothing landscape. If you are looking at a picture of a saint, sage, or religious object, you may find that it will help you create a spiritual connection. Whatever you choose, gaze at the image for a few moments, and then close your eyes and calmly try to re-create this image in your mind.

    Creative visualization. Many people meditate by visualizing an object that is not actually present. Think of something meaningful to you, and in your mind, place it on a table in a room with nothing else in it. Focus on the color, shape, texture, and smell of the object and allow your other thoughts to float away. Visualization can give your meditation a focal point and help you to calm all the chatter in your mind.

Visualize yourself in nature. One of my favorite techniques is to imagine lying in a beautiful meadow of flowers, on a deserted tropical beach, or perhaps on a mountaintop. Imagine you are staring up at white, windswept clouds, and the air is laced with the exotic essence of springtime flowers. In the distance is the soothing sound of a quiet stream.

Experience the moment. If you choose to meditate outdoors, you will experience something wonderful. Whether you are sitting in a beautiful park, resting by a waterfall, or watching a sunset, you are taking time out to enjoy the sounds, beauty, or silence of nature's soothing touch. Observe all the rich stimuli in your environment and all the sensations in your body; savor the golden moments like a precious love.

The Best Times for Meditation

The best times to meditate are at sunrise or sunset. These are the most tranquil times of the day and are very conducive to meditation. The energy during these times is in transition and holds a very sacred vibration. You may find it much easier to meditate first thing in the morning, when your mind is still fresh from sleep. At the end of the day your mind is often cluttered from daily life, so it's harder to clear your mind at this time, although doing so can be very rewarding. Nothing feels better than letting go of all your daily stress before you go to bed, and this will also assist you in having an easier time falling asleep.

If meditation at sunrise or sunset doesn't fit into your schedule, then find a time that does. It's your own personal journey, so you need to find a time that works best for you. You may be a lunchtime meditator, or maybe early evening works best for you. Whatever works, go for it—the experience is well worth your effort and energy.

SITTING STILL FOR HOW LONG?

As a beginner, you may find that you can't sit still for very long and your mind starts wandering after a few minutes. If you feel uncomfortable, if your meditation practice is unproductive, or if it is starting to frustrate you, stop for a while and try again later. Remember, you are trying to cultivate peace and focus, not stress and tension, so let it come naturally.

When you first start meditating, try to set aside just five minutes or so. Try gradually working up to 20 minutes to half an hour in each sitting. Again, don't force it; find an amount of time that works best for you.

A TYPICAL MEDITATOR IN TRAINING

For most of us the nature of the untrained mind is to wander off in different directions, like a young child will wander off and get into trouble. If you are new to meditation, your mind will wander quite often, and you have to calmly refocus onto the subject of attention. What might be going on in your head at first is something like this:

"Hey, I'm meditating—oops, here comes another thought!" Time passes and you are in tune with your breath and start to practice concepts of meditation, then all of a sudden: "Oh, no! Another thought and my nose itches, too!" You start meditating again and all of a sudden, "Hey I wonder what the surfing is like in Bali today, and I really miss that Thai food."

If this happens, don't worry: after every break in the flow, just calmly guide your focus back to your area of attention. No matter what happens, keep trying, and eventually meditation will come more easily.

Meditation Exercises

I have listed below two step-by-step guides to get you started on your journey. The first exercise is a basic meditation exercise of visualization to help you release stress and tension and enhance your mental state of mind. The second exercise is designed to focus your meditation energy toward a specific object or subject.

PERSONAL MEDITATION I

1. **Choosing a Meditation Posture.** Choose a comfortable yoga seated posture, such as kneeling pose (Thunderbolt), basic cross-legged, Perfect Posture (*Siddhasana*), or half and full lotus (*Padamasana*). Refer to Chapter 4 for details on these postures.

2. **Embracing Relaxation and Yoga Breathing.** Start breathing through your nose as slow and deep as you can, bringing your focus to your breath so your mind begins to relax. Make yourself comfortable, think passive thoughts, and try to let go of tension in your mind. Completely fill your lungs on inhalations and completely empty your lungs on exhalations. Now incorporate your *ujjayi*-controlled sound breathing, gently squeezing the air with your throat muscles, allowing yourself the control of duration on inhalation and exhalation. Let the sound itself soothe your mind. Maintain your slow deep breathing rhythm for at least 10–15 complete breaths.

3. **Practicing Sense Withdrawal.** Turn your thoughts inward and block out any distractions. This is a major part of the controlled discipline of yoga practice. Try to focus your external thoughts by bringing attention to your posture, breathing, and passive attitude.

4. **Progressive Relaxation.** Visulize different areas of your body, starting at your feet and progressing toward your head. Try to suggest relaxation to each specific body area. Try to connect your breathing with your progressive relaxation: as you exhale, isolate each area of your body and visualize it in a relaxed state.

5. **Concentration.** Visualize a flower that appeals to you; explore every aspect of this plant, including its texture, color, fragrance, and beauty. Try to recapture this flower in your mind. If the picture fades and other thoughts enter, this is completely normal; relax and return your attention to the flower. Start at the roots of the flowering plant and try to mentally touch the roots in every detail within your mind. Bring your attention up to the stem of the plant; notice the texture. Turn your attention toward the leaves and notice all the veins running through the leaves. Mentally move to the flower in full bloom, be aware of the beautiful colors, smell its essence and touch the delicate, velvety petals with your mind.

6. **Meditation (Visual).** Allow your thoughts of the flower to fade and visualize yourself seated in a meadow full of springtime flowers. Listen to your quiet breathing and imagine the softness of the warm evening sun shining gently on your back. Smell the passionate fragrance of springtime flowers riding the soft evening breeze. Bring your thoughts back to the flower and realize that you, the flower, and the whole universe are part of the same energy. Still your mind, quiet your focus, and enjoy some moments of peace.

7. Calmly travel this path as long as you like. When you are finished, relax, clear your mind, and sit quietly for another 10 slow deep breaths. When finished lay on your back and relax for a few more minutes, then slowly return to your activities.

SPECIFIC MEDITATION 2

In this meditation you are focusing your attention toward a specific object, thought, idea, or area. For this exercise you first need to follow steps 1–4 for the Personal Meditation, then follow the instructions listed below for the Specific Meditation.

5. Focus your attention onto your specific area of attention and recognize the concept, object, or problem. Make yourself very familiar with the whole concept, problem, or object, as long as you stay calm and focused. Think around the outer edges of this concept, then narrow your field to encompass the core.

6. Try to realize what you want to achieve with this concept or idea. If it is a problem, then strive to seek the actual cause of the problem. Continue to focus on this subject in a relaxed manor with your slow quiet breathing. Visualize yourself as an outside observer, nonattached to any personal or emotional waves.

7. Next, try to find a solution for the problem, or a way to improve your concept or idea. Strive to focus on all aspects of this improvement or solution. Allow your thoughts to come naturally, and flow with the rhythm of your breath. Start with a broad or general field of thought, then gradually narrow your meditation to the core issue.

8. Now you can decide how to put your solution, or improvement, into motion. Once again seek all areas for a plan on how to put your positive solution into action. Calmly review your plan of action and sit quietly with your breath. Keep your emotions separate and be an observer of your mind.

9. When finished, clear your mind and sit calmly for another 10 slow complete breaths, then lie down on your back for a few minutes, clear your mind, and relax, then go slowly back to your normal routine.

Moving Meditation: The Ultimate Yoga Practice Flow

A Moving Meditation can be achieved during any movement, such as walking, or during yoga posture practice. Yoga postures practiced as a moving meditation can create the ultimate yoga experience, which embraces both the soothing touch of softness and the powerful energy of strength.

The ultimate in Sadhana Yoga *asana* practice is to embrace all your connecting movements as a moving meditation. As you gain confidence, strength, and greater awareness, you will strive toward having a pure mind-body focus in all aspects of your movements with effortless fluidity and grace. Your practice will float like a cloud, directed by the energy of the wind. At this point you will let your mind flow free, visualizing where you are going with your movements, as your body follows your mind's lead with effortless silence.

WALKING MEDITATION—EXERCISE 3

To get the most out of this wonderful experience you might first try this walking meditation with a friend for moral support. Find a place to walk and then follow a few simple rules: no talking, and try to embrace Action Without Attachment.

1. Start walking, while beginning your yoga breathing. Strive to embrace every aspect of your breath.

2. Be totally aware of every sound, sight, and smell. Petend you are a small child and have never been out of the house. Experience each moment as if this were your last day on Earth. Find pleasure like never before from the scent of a flower, be thrilled at the sight of an unusual car, or find detail within unique people, or animals.

3. After 30 to 40 minutes, return home and sit down and try to recall some things you experienced and how you felt without talking. Notice if you were aware of your own body and mind, not just outward stimulation. When finished, take some notes and then another day give the Meditation Walk another try. Strive to be aware of every aspect of your own body and mind, yet totally aware of all that is going on around you, and at the same time be relaxed and at peace.

FUELING YOUR BODY
FOR A NATURAL
ENERGY FLOW

Food from the gods
Touch the wealth of your soul
Sacred is the body
That can never grow old

Yoga practice without proper nutrition is like trying to drive your car without the right

fuel: while it might work, you can't expect it to run at its best! Most people today treat

their bodies badly when it comes to what they eat. They fill their "tank" with most any-

thing, as long as it tastes good. This is largely due to lack of proper education on nutri-

tion, loss of our natural instincts, food cost, peer pressure, and availability.

The diet I teach in this book is a progression toward the diet used by the healthiest sages and wisest spiritual teachers of the past. All those who follow this diet will experience enlightened spiritual consciousness, increased physical and mental health, and be blessed with abundant energy. Of course, your yoga practice will greatly benefit.

LAWS OF NATURE AND YOUR NUTRITION

I am a firm believer in the philosophy "Health is truly the only real wealth." The importance of proper nutrition is one of the most valuable aspects of your Sadhana Yoga program. Without proper nutrition, you're not going to reach your full potential.

Humans are for the most part in the dark when it comes to nutrition. Through time modern men and women have drifted away from nature and therefore lost their natural instincts for eating. Instead, we rely almost entirely on marketing pitches to guide us: we are enticed by foods we see on television commercials, or restaurant reviews in newspapers. However, most of these foods are exactly what we don't need to eat. To get back on the right path, the solution is simple: Mother Nature knows best.

The good news is that through the Sadhana Yoga program you can reconnect yourself to the natural flow of energy and the laws of nature, at the same time restoring your vitality and health. This can be done without being totally extreme, fasting, shedding your clothes, and living under a rock on a remote mountain. You simply have to educate yourself, think sensibly about the food choices you make, and create a plan that puts this valuable aspect of your life into action.

UNDERSTANDING THE FOOD CHOICES YOU MAKE

All creatures living in the wild, untouched by human civilization, have instincts as to what to eat. Each separate species eats the food which is ideal for its anatomy, health, and well-being. Within each species, the diets of individual animals are almost identical.

Humans, on the other hand, have lost their natural instincts. All of us have basically the same needs for nutrition, and yet across the planet we have very diverse eating habits. We'll eat almost anything. The food industry knows if they put something in a colorful box, or serve it in a restaurant with a sprig of parsley, we will eat it, no questions asked! We have lost our natural instincts for the ability to make correct food choices. Without this internal guidance system we can and do choose to eat anything we want, and that freedom can be your friend or your enemy.

Unless you are a health-minded person, you are probably being tempted away from a natural, healthy diet. In order to enjoy complete health you have to supply your body with certain essential vitamins and minerals that are contained within a variety of natural foods. To create proper basic nutrition we need a specific amount of the following: proteins, fats, and carbohydrates.

The Importance of Protein

Protein builds and repairs the body's tissue. Within our body, the basic structure of each cell is made up of protein. We can get protein from plant or animal sources. Plant sources are preferable due to the high fat, cholesterol, and bacterial levels of animal products. Animal sources of protein include lean meat, dairy, eggs, and fish. Plant sources of dense proteins include nuts, seeds, beans, legumes, grains, tofu, tempeh, and spirulina (a fresh water blue-green algae and an excellent protein supplement). Other foods containing lower amounts of protein, yet still adding to the daily total are: avocado, cauliflower, collards, garlic, and kale.

The concept that we are not able to get enough protein without eating meat is a complete myth. In reality, the recommended daily allowance (RDA) of protein for the average adult is between 35 and 40 grams. If you are pregnant or breast-feeding, you may require additional protein. The average American eats about 120 grams of protein daily, or more. Excessive protein is very harmful to your body. The following is a list of protein from vegetarian sources.

VEGETARIAN PROTEIN SOURCES

FOOD SOURCE	SIZE SERVING	GRAMS PROTEIN
Almonds	6 oz.	18.6 grams
Avocados	3½ oz.	2.1 grams
Chickpeas	6 oz.	9.0 grams
Collard greens	3½ oz.	4.8 grams

FOOD SOURCE	SIZE SERVING	GRAMS PROTEIN
Garlic	3½ oz.	6.2 grams
Lentils	6 oz.	24.7 grams
Mung beans	6 oz.	24.2 grams
Peanuts	6 oz.	26.0 grams
Peas, green	3½ oz	6.3 grams
Pecans	6 oz.	9.2 grams
Rye grain	6 oz.	12.1 grams
Sesame seeds	6 oz.	18.6 grams
Soybeans	6 oz.	22.0 grams
Sunflower seeds	6 oz.	24.0 grams
Walnuts	6 oz.	14.8 grams
Wheat (winter)	6 oz.	12.3 grams

Problems Related to Excess Protein

It would be very hard not to get enough protein from a diet that included a variety of the foods mentioned above. A greater concern is getting too much protein from concentrated animal sources that are also high in cholesterol, fat, and bacteria. Excessive protein can lead to osteoporosis, weakened liver, unhealthy colon, and a variety of other serious problems.

The Importance of Fats

The fats we eat create heat and energy within our body. Sources of fats are much the same as the proteins. Animal fats are found in both meat and dairy products. Plant sources of fat include nuts, seeds, and fatty fruits like avocado, olive, and coconut. Plant sources supply a much cleaner form of fat and are free from harmful saturated fat, which produces cholesterol.

The Truth Behind Fat and Cholesterol

There are basically two kinds of fats. There are healthy fats that we call unsaturated fats, and there are unhealthy fats that we call saturated fats. Most Americans consume too much saturated fat, which is often found in mass-produced, prepackaged, or "fast" food. Saturated fats are also found in whole milk and dairy products, cheeses, and all animal products such as meats and eggs. Another source of saturated fat is heated oils, which are used to fry foods. When oils are heated, they turn into "hydrogenated fat" and have a property that allows them to coagulate or harden at room temperature. Margarine, for example, is one kind of hydrogenated fat. Hydrogenated oils cannot be digested by your body and are very destructive to your circulatory system and your overall health.

The source of the oil is unimportant in terms of whether or not it can be hydrogenated. Even cold-pressed oils become hydrogenated when heated. The worst oils to consume are coconut oil and palm kernel oil. To avoid these and all other heated oils, you need to carefully read ingredient labels on all the products you buy, and try to stay away from oily, prepared foods. This means avoiding all fried food, stir fries, and any other foods prepared in heated oils.

Studies have shown that by eating a diet high in saturated fats, one is more susceptible to having high cholesterol levels. Excessive cholesterol has been proven to be a contributing factor in hardening of the arteries, heart attacks, strokes, and some forms of cancer.

Polyunsaturated Fats

Polyunsaturated fats are considered to be healthy fats, and the foods which supply polyunsaturated fats actually help to remove the saturated fat from your body, clean out the veins, and reverse the destruction done from eating the wrong foods. Polyunsaturated fats are found in raw nuts and fatty fruits such as avocado, soybeans, and raw seeds. The highest sources of polyunsaturated fats are macadamia nuts, pine nuts, sunflower seeds, primrose oil, flax seeds, and avocados. However, if any of these items have been processed, heated, or altered in any way, then they are no longer considered to be healthy, polyunsaturated items.

One of the most popular foods to get the right amount of polyunsaturated fats is deep-water fish. However, there are many drawbacks to eating fish in today's world, mainly due to water pollution. Many sources of pollution have contributed to contaminating fish with toxic substances, including mercury. A safer way to get the same nutrients found in fish, like important omega-3 essential fatty acids, is by eating flaxseeds or using flaxseed oil. You can blend whole flaxseeds into a smoothie, glass of juice, or salad dressing. Try grinding dry flaxseed in an herb grinder or regular blender, then use on cereal. Strive to use a tablespoon or more of flaxseeds per day, or you can use flaxseed oil.

Monounsaturated Fats

Monounsaturated fats are a close cousin to polyunsaturated fats. They are also very good for you, and can be found in many healthy foods, including almonds, hazelnuts, and avocados.

The Importance of Carbohydrates

Carbohydrates supply the body with sugar in the form of glucose, which becomes a source of energy that fuels the central nervous system. Carbohydrates can be divided into two groups: simple and complex. Simple carbohydrates (glucose sugars) include sucrose (found in sugar), lactose (found in milk), and maltose (found in malt). When you take any of these refined, processed sugars into your body, they are converted into glucose extremely rapidly. This causes fluctuations in blood-sugar levels and can lead to blood-sugar problems such as diabetes.

Complex carbohydrates are natural sugars found in grains, fruits, and vegetables. Complex carbohydrates transform into sugar more slowly within your system and therefore don't give your metabolism the unhealthy "sugar jolt" of simple carbohydrates. Complex carbohydrates are also some of the best foods we can eat, because they also contain fiber, vitamins, and minerals, and are digested without the adverse effects of simple sugars. When choosing fruit, pick seeded fruit over seedless. Seedless fruit is higher in sugar and lower in nutrition.

However, too much complex carbohydrates can be detrimental to your health. If you are overweight, having mood swings, or blood-sugar problems, you should eliminate all processed simple carbohydrates and limit your grains, sweet fruits, and starchy vegetables. If you have a health problem and are concerned about carbohydrate intake, you should seek advice from your family doctor or nutritionist.

The Truth Behind Fiber

Many of us eat a low-fiber diet, which means that we eat lots of soft foods that have the fibers removed. However, fiber helps to gently brush out the intestinal tract, which can help to prevent many problems, including colon cancer. Through the years of eating the wrong foods and a diet low in fiber, you can create toxic pockets in your intestinal tract and hardened plaque on the walls of your colon, thereby creating a perfect atmosphere for sickness and disease to manifest. Adding fiber to your diet will also help to lower your cholesterol and stabilize your blood-sugar levels, as well as helping to prevent constipation and hemorrhoids.

The very best fibrous foods are fresh fruits, vegetables, seaweeds, and whole unprocessed grains. To change over to a high-fiber diet, start by adding more fresh fruit, vegetables, and whole grains to your diet. Rice bran or wheat bran (the husk, or roughage, from the outer grain) is also a good fiber-rich supplement. Psyllium and flaxseeds are gelatinous seeds that coat the intestines and help to remove unwanted particles, and although they are not high in fiber, they act as if they are.

If you base your diet on a low-cholesterol, low-fat, and high-fiber diet, you can greatly reverse all the effects of eating the wrong foods, and at the same time replenish your body with healthy living food. With correct nutrition you will keep your body healthy and strong throughout your whole life. Try to move your food choices toward more raw foods, striving for at least a combination of 70 percent raw fruits, vegetables, nuts, seeds, grains, and beans. This is what makes a healthy diet and a healthy you.

Vitamins

Vitamins assist with the body's normal metabolic functioning. All the vitamins necessary for a healthy active life can be found in fruits, vegetables, nuts, seeds, grains, seaweeds, bee pollen, and blue-green algae. The best source of natural, easily digested vitamins is through a variety of fresh squeezed, uncooked organically grown fruit and vegetable juices. Drinking juiced fruits and vegetables is a wonderful practice to get into: there are endless combinations that will please your palette, and they take only minutes to prepare. To get the most out of these juices, try drinking them thirty minutes before your meal. If you drink them with your meals the liquid may interfere with proper digestion. If you drink fresh-squeezed fruit or vegetable juice before your meals, it gives you a very concentrated source of easily digested and assimilated vitamins, as well as curbing your appetite.

Minerals

Minerals are the materials used for building tissue and serve as body regulators. They are found in abundance in organically grown fruits, vegetables, nuts, seeds, grains, and seaweed.

The recommended daily amounts of all the required vitamins and minerals can be easily supplied from plant sources.

VITAMIN AND MINERAL SOURCES

NUTRIENTS	RDA	PLANT—FOOD SOURCE
Vitamin A (beta carotene)	4,000– 5,000 IU	Carrots, vegetables
B complex	1.2-1.4 MG	Sprouts, leafy vegetables
B-1, B-2, B-3, B-6	————————	Pineapple, seaweed
Vitamin B-12	3 MCG	Spirulina, fermented foods
Vitamin C	60 MG	Citrus fruit, berries
Vitamin D	400 IU	Sunlight exposure
Vitamin E	10–20 IU	Cabbage, leafy greens
Folic Acid	400 MCG	Leafy greens, carrots
Niacin	20 MG	Rice bran, vegetables
Calcium	800 MG	Sesame seeds, kale
Phosphorus	800 MG	Lentils, pinto beans
Magnesium	300–500 MG	Dark green vegetables
Iodine	150 MCG	Kelp, pineapple, greens
Iron	10–18 MG	Cherries, apricots, prunes
Zinc	15 MG	Soybeans, spinach

Supplementing Your Vitamins and Minerals

Vitamins and food supplements can compliment a good balanced diet, but are not a replacement. If you have adopted a natural healthy vitamin-rich diet, and think you might still be lacking a specific recommended amount of a particular vitamin, you can supplement your diet with isolated vitamins in pill form. There are basically two forms of vitamin supplements: water-soluble and fat-soluble. The fat-soluble vitamins (Vitamins A, D, E) are stored in the body, so it is possible that you can build up an excess amount. Caution should be taken not to use too much of these supplements. Water-soluble vitamins (Vitamins C and B) are largely excreted and are not stored in appreciable amounts in the body.

Super Food Supplements

In addition to isolated vitamins there are supplemental super foods found in health-food stores that can add important vitamins and minerals to your diet. Many of these "super supplements" can complete your daily requirements for a variety of different needs. As with all vitamin supplements, these super supplements are better assimilated when taken with meals, rather than on an empty stomach. When shopping for vitamins, buy an organic-based food-source vitamin.

Bee pollen: is rich in B vitamins, protein, and many amino acids. It helps your muscles increase their strength and endurance. Many athletes use bee pollen before and after their workouts. The proper daily dosage of bee pollen is a tablespoon taken every other day. Bee pollen comes in powdered form, or capsules so that you can ingest it in a variety of ways: you can blend it into your drinks or eat it straight from a spoon. You can put it on your cereal, salads, or even make it into an energy bar by mixing it with dried fruits and squeezing the mixture together. However, some people are allergic to bee pollen, so it is good to test yourself with small doses. Try a quarter of a teaspoon, and if you don't have any adverse reaction, then gradually build up to the recommended dosage.

Spirulina and blue-green algae: These two names both refer to nutritious freshwater algae. If you could pick any food to take to a deserted island, spirulina or blue-green algae would be the one to take. These supplemental food sources are rich in vitamins and a good source of essential amino acids. Blue-green algae is also very high in protein and chlorophyll, as well as high in vitamin B12. Spirulina and blue-green algae are composed of about 70 percent protein, which can help you to reduce your blood-sugar levels.

Kelp and other seaweeds: are high in many of the major minerals and B vitamins. You will also find potassium, iron, calcium, and magnesium within seaweeds. Seaweeds can also be used as a very tasty seasoning. You can use seaweeds in soups, salads, and sandwiches. A few examples of very nutritional seaweeds are Dulse, Nori, Arame, and Hijiki.

Kelp is very high in iodine, and along with other seaweeds has the unique ability to help to remove radioactive particles and heavy metals from the body. Those of us who live in cities are exposed to radioactive particles and heavy metals on a daily basis.

Wheat grass: is one of the healthiest plant foods available. Wheat grass is one of the richest sources of chlorophyll, which acts as a protective element against pollution of environment and radiation. Wheat grass also works as a wonderful blood purifier, has anti-aging properties, and is a high-energy food with fair amounts of protein, and rich in vitamins and minerals.

Wheat grass is most effective in juice form. The dried variety has very minimal effect as opposed to the fresh. Go to your local health-food store or juice bar and ask them for fresh-juiced wheat grass. One or two ounces of wheat grass juice every other day is excellent for your health. A few ounces of wheat grass is equivalent to eating twenty or thirty organic salads.

TRAVELING THE PATH TO A HEALTHY DIET

There is more than one path to attain good health through nutrition. Yet among all other aspects, vegetarianism has proved to be a valuable asset to good health. Vegetarians do not eat meat, fish, or poultry. A vegan is a vegetarian who also excludes dairy products. As you can guess, I support a totally vegetarian diet, although that may seem a bit extreme for you. Not only will you become healthier, you will be practicing the yogic ideal of *ahimsa*, or nonviolence toward animals.

The Science Behind a Vegetarian Diet

Nature often gives us warning signals, but we tend to listen to our doctors. Now, members of the National Cancer Institute report that heavy meat eating is related to high incidence of all types of cancer. Societies which are mostly vegetarian have 80 percent less chance of getting cancer than meat-eating societies. Many other studies have proven that those who base their diet on meat are at high risk for heart attack, stroke, and artery disease. Living parasites are also commonly found in those who eat meat on a regular basis.

At one time fish and seafood could have been considered a healthful addition to the diet. However, due to a general lack of respect for nature, many of our ponds, lakes, streams, rivers, and coastal waters are polluted. Therefore, many experts agree it is no longer recommended to eat fish and seafood as a healthy part of good nutrition, unless you are absolutely sure where these foods came from and had them tested for toxins before eating.

Six Simple Rules to Enhance Your Overall Health

The following six rules are the backbone of a true yogic diet. To begin to make a change, choose one of these rules and master it. Then try to apply a second, and third. Soon you will be eating and feeling much better. However, no matter which rule you begin with, try not to replace your current diet by overeating any of the good foods mentioned above. Overeating is hard on digestion and can be unhealthy for you, even if you are eating healthy natural food.

1. **Base your diet on vegetarian foods**—cut back on meat and other animal products, including eggs and dairy products as well. Eat more fresh, raw, steamed, and baked vegetables. Strive for a diet free from all animal products; many experts in the field of nutrition will agree that you do not need any animal products to be completely healthy.

2. **Eat a variety of foods**—don't eat the same thing every day. A variety of fruits and vegetables, nuts and seeds, supply a vast array of healthy vitamins, minerals, and essential amino acids.

3. **Reduce the fat** content in your body, stay away from saturated fats and heated oils. Try to avoid fried foods whenever possible.

4. **Increase fiber** in your diet by eating more fresh raw fruits and vegetables and whole grains.

5. **Eat organically grown foods.** Commercially grown food is loaded with chemical pesticides, which are not good for your health or the environment.

6. **Eat more plant food in its natural state.** Put more fresh raw foods in your diet. Try to eat whole unprocessed foods. Foods in their whole natural state retain all of the healthy natural fats, carbohydrates, proteins, living enzymes, vitamins, and minerals as contained in nature.

Now that you know why you should incorporate a healthy diet and have some basic guidelines, all you have to do is get motivated and create a change for the better. Getting started on a new diet is both exciting and yet a bit scary. You are already learning how to embrace a new kind of yoga workout program. I think of my nutrition program as an extension of Sadhana Yoga, and you should, too. Just as you practiced the first breath and posture on your yoga mat, and then moved blissfully into relaxation and meditation, now, by choosing to adopt a healthier diet, you are taking one more step toward achieving great thoughts into action and resulting in better health. You'll find that getting started on a new eating regimen is simply a four-step process:

Step One—Planting Positive Thoughts

Choosing to begin a better diet and getting started on a new program of nutrition is the only thing keeping you from walking the path. Thoughts are seeds, and if you plant some positive thoughts along the lines of a healthier diet, then these seeds will grow into positive action. Set some time aside, sit down in a quiet place, and define your nutrition goals. Do some deep breathing and practice a bit of yoga to enhance your self-confidence. Taking on one new concept is already a major step toward a better life for you and all those you come into contact with.

Step Two—Building the Foundation

Check the Resources section for suggestions of books on health and nutrition. Using those as a guide, make a list of what you need for your new improved diet. Now locate a grocery or health-food shop which carries organic natural food. Many supermarkets now have health-food sections and a large line of organic produce. The cost for natural healthy food may be a bit higher than commercially grown, yet in the long run you will save money with your good health. Look for healthy alternatives for foods you enjoy and stock your house with healthy food for your new diet. See the shopping list at the end of this chapter for some great pantry ideas.

Step Three—Moving into Action

Put your thoughts and new foods to use by adopting your own level of my healthy diet listed in this chapter. Start by substituting one or two healthy meals for your usual meal. The best inspiration is to consciously think about what you are eating before you eat. Think about where this food came from and what effect it has on your physical and mental body. After a week or so, gradually add more healthy meals until you have eventually upgraded your whole menu.

Step Four—Detoxify Your Body with Diet and Juice Fasting

Fasting is a method of helping the body to naturally cleanse itself of stored impurities, toxins, and waste, along with giving the digestive system a well-needed rest. By avoiding certain foods, eating sparingly, and at certain times avoiding solid food, you are giving your body a cleansing which helps to improve the function of your vital organs and creates enhanced condition of overall health.

The Science Behind Fasting

All of us have consumed toxins and pollutants through the food that we eat, and we have also been exposed to overall pollution of our environment. A portion of these foreign unhealthy substances are stored in our body. Fasting is one of the best ways to help eliminate many of the toxins. Fasting also cleanses the body of excess mucus, stored chemicals, and drugs that may distract from your health, vitality, and longevity. Many people take a fast for the sole purpose of losing weight. This is not a recommended fasting practice, and should not be done without the correct supervision from your medical practitioner. In addition, if you do not improve your base diet, chances are you will gain all the weight back.

WHAT HAPPENS TO YOUR BODY DURING A FAST?

During a fast your body metabolism has a built-in response to begin searching every part of your anatomy for unwanted toxins and weakened or diseased cells and then removes them from your bloodstream. There are five avenues for elimination: lungs, kidneys, bowels, mouth, nose, and skin. In a healthy body all these avenues of elimination are allowed to operate freely. If any one of these avenues is blocked, your health will be compromised. It is not healthy, natural, or advantageous to restrict toxins from being eliminated from your body. During a fast, or restricted cleansing diet, all these avenues of elimination in your body are greatly enhanced and will assist to create an easy elimination of toxins from your body.

FIVE AVENUES TO ELIMINATE BODY TOXINS:

(1)—Lungs (through exhalation).

(2)—Kidneys (through urination).

(3)—Bowels (through stool).

(4)—Skin (through sweating).

(5)—Nose and Mouth (through mucus discharge).

Types of Detoxifying Fasts

There are three types of cleansing fasts. Choose one of the following methods which is best suited to your own needs. It is advisable to start your cleansing by washing the impurities out of your colon through the use of an enema, or colonic. You can do an enema at home with ½ gallon of warm water, or look up colon therapist in your phone book. This will greatly assist in the cleansing process. Also, if you have a blood-sugar problem, dilute your fruit juices 50 percent with bottled water, or substitute fresh-squeezed, green vegetable juice such as celery, cucumber, lettuce, or kale. Blood-sugar problems would also benefit from supplementing your cleansing with blue-green algae or spirulina.

(A)—*Light Cleansing*: This cleansing is ideal for those who have a poor diet and little or no experience with body detoxification. This cleansing restricts your diet to raw uncooked fruits and dark green leafy vegetables. If you have blood-sugar problems, skip the sweet fruit and substitute cucumbers. A sample light cleansing would mean having seeded fruit for breakfast, raw salad with lemon and avocado for lunch, and herbal tea or fresh-squeezed juice for dinner, with no restrictions between meals on bottled water and more fresh-squeezed juices. Continue this program for 1 to 7 days. Then break your cleansing with some lightly steamed vegetables for a few days, then take the steps to adopt a healthy diet.

(B)—*Moderate Cleansing*: For those who are predominately vegetarian and have tried body detoxification in the past. A moderate cleansing removes solid food from the diet, so that you are eating only raw, blended uncooked seeded fruits and fresh raw blended vegetables (you can use the juice instead), adding lots of green leaf vegetable juice. A sample moderate cleansing would mean drinking fresh squeezed vegetable juices for breakfast, fresh juicy fruit, blended with leafy greens and apple, for lunch (staying away from seedless fruit, which is higher in sugar and lower in nutrition), and an herbal tea for dinner. Continue this program from 1 to 5 days, and then you can break the cleansing by first adding raw salads and fresh fruits. Then the next day add blended nuts or raw nut butters to your salad and fruit. Then gradually adopt a healthy regular eating program.

(C)—*Heavy Cleansing*: This cleansing is best suited for those who are already vegetarians and striving to become vegans and eat at least 70 percent raw food in their diet. A heavy cleansing is considered to be a true fast. It restricts the intake of all solid food, drinking only fresh-squeezed diluted fruit and vegetable juices, green drinks, filtered water, and herb teas (green drinks are made of the juice extracted from fresh, raw, green chlorophyll-rich vegetables, such as: celery, cucumber, spinach, lettuce, kale, parsley and collard greens). A sample heavy cleansing would mean beginning your day with 50 percent diluted fruit juice, and for lunch having diluted vegetable juice with mostly juice of leafy greens. Finish the day with an herbal tea for dinner. Continue this program from 1 to 5 days. When finished break your fast with juicy seeded fruit, or raw salad, then gradually return to a healthy eating program. If you have blood-sugar problems, use cucumber instead of sweet fruit.

Remember that the addition of any cooked food, protein, or starch will completely stop the toxin elimination and you will no longer be in a cleansing body detoxification. During the fast, your body will rest, cleanse, rejuvenate, and try to heal your whole system naturally. For best results, it is most appropriate to pick a time when you can rest, or at least cut your work and stress load down greatly. Practice light yoga and take moderate walks. At night relax in a warm Epsom salt bath.

You can safely fast or maintain a restricted diet for 1 to 3 days. If you are more experienced you can fast up to 5 or 6 days. A fast of longer than this is not advisable without supervision of a doctor or licensed professional.

Preparing to Fast

It is best to first change your diet before you begin a fast, so your body doesn't go into shock. Slowly move away from processed food, junk food, and meat and animal products and introduce more raw and cooked fruits and vegetables, nuts, seeds, and grain, and fresh fruit and vegetable juices. After a few weeks of an improved diet, you can try to fast from anywhere from two to four days.

It is best to start and finish your fast with an enema, or colonic. During your fast your intestines will become loaded with poisons from the body as your system is trying to eliminate these toxins. An enema or colonic will greatly assist in removing this waste from your colon much quicker than your normal metabolic function can and therefore leave you feeling very refreshed.

The Emotional Response to Fasting

The second limb of the eight-limbed yogic path to enlightenment pertains to ethics and morals: in particular, only hard work and effort builds paradise. You cannot achieve health by having it handed to you. The Sanskrit word *tapas* is translated as meaning an effort or burning, which involves self-discipline, purification, and austerity. The word *austerity* in this context means to work at something whereby there is an exchange between discomfort and attaining a positive goal. *Tapas* then means to undergo some physical and mental discomfort in order to achieve enhanced physical and mental health. While many of us want an instant cure, without any lack of energy, or change in bad habits, it is not possible!

Fasting can be very hard work, depending on the level of toxins in your body. While your body is eliminating toxins, you will experience days when you feel dizzy and weak, and other days you will feel on top of the world. It is best to avoid extensive physical and mental stress during your fast. When fasting, your energy level will be lower and your emotions a little more fragile and delicate. Some people have more energy during the fast, and others will be weak, drained, and emotionally fragile. The slight discomfort is a small price to pay for a clean bill of health.

Breaking Your Fast

If you begin your fast and feel like you cannot or do not want to go the distance, simply break your fast by eating sensibly. Your first meal should be a leafy green salad without dressing, or fresh juicy seeded fruits.

The first few days following a successful fast should consist of meals that have a laxative or cleansing effect, rather than quickly rebuilding your diet. The reason for this is that it is very important to quickly eliminate the toxins that have been stored up throughout the body as a result of the fasting or cleansing. Never break a fast with high-protein foods like nuts, seeds, greens, beans, meat, or dairy products. Never break your fast with starchy foods like potatoes, yams, pasta, or bananas. Instead try raw salad or fresh fruit; the next meal could be lightly steamed vegetables or different vegetables with avocado.

I like to call my eating plan the Diet That Loves You Most. It has four levels so that you can gradually incorporate this diet into your lifestyle. We are all at different stages of evolution in our diets. Some people can change very easily, while others will have to make a gradual change over a longer period of time.

My diet comprises mostly *sattvic* foods. In traditional yoga philosophy, all foods fall into one of three main categories:

Sattvic **Food**—Healthy, wholesome, nourishing food. *Sattvic* food supplies your body with all ingredients necessary for a healthy active life. These foods include fresh raw fruits, vegetables, sprouts, nuts, seeds, grains, and seaweed.

Rajasic **Food**—This is food that unnaturally stimulates your body, causing you to "run" way beyond your normal capabilities. These foods will overtax your system, which can cause much strain and depletion to both your mental and physical health, leading to a lack of energy, mood swings, and an overall weakened immune system. A sample of these foods include coffee, sugar, fructose, and herbs such as yohimbi and ma huang. Through the yogic tradition garlic, onions, and spicy foods are placed in this category, only because they tend to unsettle the mind. Garlic, onions, and cayenne pepper are very healthy foods.

Tamasic **Food**—This is just plain unhealthy food; eating this kind of food detracts from your health and creates an environment for sickness and disease. These foods include junk food, highly processed food, commercially treated foods, sugar, white flour products, non-organically grown food, fried food, high-fat food, excess meat, dairy products, and eggs.

Four Levels of Diet and Nutritional Habits:

To begin, first choose the level which best accommodates your own present eating habits. Be honest with yourself: it is better to make small accomplishments successfully than to try something grand and totally crash and burn. Small success builds self-confidence for greater accomplishments later on.

Level 1 Student

This level caters to those who are new with the concept of eating healthy and have not restricted their eating habits. The typical Level I student is still eating red meat and dairy products and is not restricting foods that are high in cholesterol or fat, or are low in fiber. Fruits and vegetables are not comprising much of your current diet, which probably still consists of 80 percent or more cooked food, with no restrictions on coffee, soft drinks, sugar, salt, junk food, or candy.

Instant Help for Level 1 Students

The first thing Level I students should do is add more fiber-rich products to their daily meals and cut down on fat. Become more aware of the foods you eat, making an effort to avoid less-nutritious, vitamin-depleted, and/or processed foods. Try to use healthier substitutes for meat and dairy whenever possible: choose organically raised leaner cuts of beef, and get into the habit of removing all visible fat on meats before cooking. Switch from high-fat dairy products to organic low-fat cheeses, yogurts, and milk, or try to substitute rice or soy milk for dairy milk. Try a vegetarian meal now and then. Strive to add more fruit and vegetables into your daily intake. Try to add more raw fruits and vegetables to your meals, and drink plenty of water and fresh juices daily. Avoid overeating: eat to live, don't live to eat.

Level 2 Student

Level 2 is appropriate for students who have some knowledge and practice in healthy eating principals. These students are already trying to cut down on their intake of meat and dairy products, and can now make a greater effort to maintain a low-cholesterol, low-fat diet. In fact, 30 to 40 percent of their diet is already comprised of raw foods. They have tried a vegetarian meal now and then, and often substitute nondairy products for dairy products. This level person has made an effort to restrict coffee, soft drinks, sugar, salt, junk food, and candy.

Instant Help for Level 2 Students

All the suggestions from Level 1 still apply, but you can now progress a little further toward a healthier diet. You are very interested in moving toward a vegetarian diet and realize the benefits as you add more plant foods to each meal. You would like your diet to include 60 to 70 percent from plant sources such as fruits, vegetables, nuts, seeds and grains. Drink vegetable juice and juices made from green, leafy vegetables on a regular basis. Try to eat more organically grown foods. Take time to relax when you eat, and read books on health and nutrition listed in the Resources section.

Level 3 Student

This level is for someone who is already following a primarily vegetarian diet. They might eat meat only on occasion, and are very familiar with healthy diet principals and practice them on a regular basis. While they still may use dairy products, they often substitute nondairy alternatives, like soy cheeses or soy milk. They try to eat a low-fat, low-cholesterol diet and include plenty of fiber. Over 50 percent of their diet is from fruits and vegetables, with a high concentration of completely raw meals, like salads. They rarely eat sugar, salt, candy, or junk food. Level 3 students might shop regularly at the health-food store for healthier substitutes to common, though less nutritious foods. They try to always eat organically grown foods and have thought about doing a juice fast or raw-food cleansing diet.

Instant Help for Level 3 Students

All the suggestions from Levels 1 and 2 would still apply. In addition, try to completely eliminate dairy products from your diet, use more nut milks, seed cheeses, and nondairy frozen desserts. Add more dark leafy greens and sprouts to your meals whenever possible and drink fresh squeezed juices daily. Strive for a diet of 60 to 70 percent raw uncooked plant food. Buy only organically grown food, fast one to three days a few times every year. Read books on health and teach others in need.

Level 4 Student

This level is the most strict, and is for those who are striving toward a spiritual high-energy diet. These students already have extensive knowledge on the principals of health, diet, and lifestyle, and practice these principals on a regular basis. Their diet is totally vegan, completely devoid of all meat and dairy products. Raw uncooked food now compromises at least 70 percent of their daily food intake, though they are striving for an all-raw food diet. Level 4 students eat plenty of sprouts, indoor greens (like sprouted buckwheat greens, sunflower greens) and use sprouted nuts and grains on a regular basis. The Level 4 student drinks fresh-squeezed rich green drinks and wheat grass daily, and on numerous occasions has tried a strict cleansing diet and juice fast. (Green drinks are made of the juice extracted from fresh, raw, green chlorophyll-rich vegetables, such as: celery, cucumber, spinach, lettuce, kale, parsley, and collards).

Instant Help for Level 4 Students

All suggestions from Levels 1, 2, and 3 would still apply. In addition, strive toward a diet of 80 to 100 percent raw fruits, vegetables, sprouts, indoor greens, sprouted nuts, seeds, and grains in a ratio of 50–60 percent vegetables, 20 percent fruits, 10 percent starch, 10 percent protein, including raw natural fats from plant sources. Seek to have simple meals with few combinations and search for edible wild food whenever possible. Make a meal of wild berries and dandelion greens. Strive to fast five days three times a year. Eat only two meals a day and try to eat only organically grown food. Teach others about the healing benefits of a high-energy, very nutritious raw foods. Be kind and compassionate, extend your heart into your actions. Spend time with nature, read, write, and become a part of nature's infinite energy. Always be ready to learn and support other positive ideas whenever you can.

The Path to the Diet That Loves You Most

After changing what you eat you will notice your body acting much more favorably toward the natural living foods, thereby inspiring you to substitute more and more nutritionally complete foods for depleted, processed foods. By combining the diet, fitness, and health habits I've suggested throughout this book, you will cleanse your body of toxins, then rebuild with proper nutrition, fresh air, and regular exercise.

Basic Tips for All Levels of Nutrition:

These basic rules will help guide all levels a step toward the diet that loves you most. Whether you are a newcomer to the idea of changing your diet, or someone with more experience, you will find the following tips of value.

Take your time—When transcending to a healthier diet, go slowly. Fast changes are very difficult and can often cause very uncomfortable cleansing reactions within your body. Many of these reactions can be avoided by taking your time and simply alternating cleansing with healthy rebuilding, plus cleansing your colon with enemas and colonics. Cleansing reactions can be in the form of skin blemishes or rash, stuffy nose, headache, dizziness, fever, and lack of energy and ability to concentrate. Progress can be seen within a few weeks, yet don't expect miracles overnight: a lifetime of unhealthy diet and lifestyle cannot be corrected in a few days or weeks. With daily effort the end result of physical and mental health is well worth your energy and effort.

Hydrate your body—Drink plenty of water daily to keep you well hydrated and better able to thoroughly flush toxins from your body. It is always better to drink more rather than less, especially in the summer, when you lose fluids through sweating. Strive for drinking at least eight glasses of water daily. Try to choose bottled water, preferably distilled, or springwater. You can drink water at any temperature, and you may use herbal teas as well.

Be kind to yourself—and allow some splurge days now and then. Talk to likeminded people, read, study, and practice healthy diet and living. Educate yourself and visualize the many benefits of an improved diet and lifestyle. Think positive thoughts, be confident, and take positive action to fulfill your goals. Most of all be happy, keeping your sense of humor. You are doing a wonderful thing not only for yourself but for all those around you and future generations. What is healthy for you is also healthy for the whole planet. Inner harmony creates outer harmony and we all benefit.

Eat to live—don't live to eat—Eat when you are truly hungry, not just for fun, pleasure, or to cover up stress. At mealtime eat slowly and focus on calm, relaxing, and comfortable ideas. Avoid watching TV or working on your computer while eating. Use portion control, and try to eat enough food yet without feeling uncomfortable. If possible rest and relax for a few minutes after your meal. In relationship to yoga exercise, try to allow at least an hour after a moderate meal before practice, and allow two hours or more after a heavy meal. Ideally do yoga on an empty stomach, or prior to your practice drink a blended protein smoothie or fresh-squeezed vegetable juice.

FOOD COMBINING MADE SIMPLE

When graduating to a diet that includes more raw foods, you will experience some occasional digestive problems from mixing raw food with cooked food. Always eat raw food first, as it will digest more quickly. If you have a problem chewing raw food, simply blend it up for easier digestion. This helps to break down the fiber without losing nutritional value due to cooking. You can make raw smoothies, blended hot soups, or dips and spreads.

You can make life much easier on your digestive system by simply observing the concepts of food-combining. There are four standard food-combining groups: fruits, vegetables, proteins, and starches.

FRUITS

Fruits digest the quickest and therefore should be eaten before other foods. Dried fruits and bananas require a bit longer to digest: bananas are a bit heavier than most fruits, and mildly starchy and dried fruit is very concentrated, especially if it has not been soaked to reconstitute. Fruits combine best with other fruits of the same variety, such as: acid fruits (like citrus), sub-acid fruits (like apples and pears), and sweet fruits (figs, persimmons, and bananas). In the winter dried fruits or sub-acid fruits may be eaten with nuts. However, it is always best to reconstitute the dried fruit first.

VEGETABLES

Vegetables take a little bit longer to digest than fruits; however, if they are eaten raw, the digestion time is considerably less than a cooked version. Vegetables combine best with other vegetables, or with proteins or starches. I have found from experience raw vegetables and fruits mix well together, especially if juiced or blended.

STARCHES

Starches are grains, potatoes, and winter squashes. Beans and legumes are often considered a starch, but only when they are raw or sprouted. Starches combine best with vegetables or other starches. Cooked starches take a long time to digest, and if they are followed by fresh fruit the starch actually ferments in the intestine and can cause much discomfort. Try not to mix proteins and starches at the same meal, because this will slow down the digestive process.

PROTEINS

Proteins take the longest to digest, especially if you are eating animal proteins. Raw nuts and seeds take about four hours to digest, whereas meat can take twelve hours or longer. Proteins combine best with vegetables or other proteins.

FOOD COMBINING

If your diet is mostly raw food, you can generally mix most fruits and vegetables. Nuts and seeds are a little more dense yet can be eaten with all vegetables or many fruits in any order without having any digestive problems, especially if they are blended together. A lot of food combining is attributed to the water content of various different foods. Watermelon, for example, is very high-water-content fruit which digests much quicker than nuts, so you would not want to eat these foods at the same meal.

HEALTHY SHOPPING LIST

The following items can be found in a health-food store or the health-food section at your local grocery:

Almond butter—Almonds ground into smooth paste, like peanut butter, yet easier to digest (choose raw, not roasted).

Almond milk—Milk-like substance made from almonds. Has no animal products, will not cause hardening of the arteries, and tastes great. Blend ⅓ cup almonds with 10 ounces water or juice, add 1 banana for a shake.

Bread (sprouted)—Bread made from sprouted grains which is both higher in fiber and lower in gluten. Comes in a variety of types, and brands. Manna or Essene are two brands of naturally sweet, flourless, whole grain, unleavened bread.

Burger buns, or hot dog buns (sprouted)—Buns made from sprouted grains, higher in nutrition, fiber, and lower in gluten.

Carob—Healthy substitute for cocoa, a bean of the carob tree. Regular chocolate is high in caffeine, fat, and sugar. Carob powder can be used in baking, drinks and candies.

Cashew milk—Healthy protein drink with no animal products. Blend ⅓ cup cashews with 10 ounces water or juice, add 1 banana for a shake.

Cereal (whole grain)—Try to buy whole grain cereal which is not highly processed, and refined, with added sugar. Use whole grain, cracked grain, or rolled oats, wheat, rye, barley.

Cheese (nondairy)—There are a number of brands of nondairy cheese which taste just like cheese and can be used in cooking. These cheeses will not affect your cholesterol levels, or artery blockage, as does the traditional dairy variety.

Dolmas—stuffed with brown rice, Grape leaves found in the deli section of natural-food stores.

Dulse—Type of seaweed, used in salads and cooking, high in calcium, B-vitamins, iodine and minerals from the sea.

Egg replacer (vegetable product)—This egg replacer is made from tapioca beans and is a healthy substitute for eggs, which are high in fat. You can use this in any recipe to replace eggs.

Egg salad (mock)—Made from soybeans, tastes like egg salad, only higher in nutrition and without the fat.

Fakin' Bacon—A healthy vegetarian low-fat meat substitute, tastes like bacon yet contains no animal products.

Flaxseeds—Nutritious seed contains the essential fatty oils necessary for good health. Blend in soups, drinks, salads, dressings, or sprinkle on cereal.

Fresh produce—Organically grown raw fruits and vegetables high in fiber, with elements to assist in cleansing and building a healthy body. Stock up on leafy greens for juicing; these greens contain high amounts of chlorophyll, which help to protect your body against pollution of environment. Strive to stay away from too much seedless fruit; it is higher in sugar and lower in nutrition.

Grains—Buy whole unprocessed organically grown grains. Try a variety such as wheat, rye, kamut, spelt, millet, amaranth, quinoa, and buckwheat.

Herbal teas—Choose herbal teas without caffeine and use freely hot or cold to replace high-sugar processed drinks.

Honey (raw)—Choose raw, unheated, unfiltered honey as a sweetener for drinks, cereal, baking, and in making natural desserts.

Ice cream (nondairy)—You will find a number of great products like Rice Dream and Ice Bean, which are made from rice and soybeans and come in a variety of tasty flavors.

Juice—Try to make your own juice. If you have to buy pre-made juice, choose juice which is made from organically grown produce, without concentrates, no sugar, no fructose, just fresh juice.

Liquid aminos (Paul Braggs)—A low sodium healthy substitute for soy sauce, helps supply essential aminos. Use on salads, sandwiches, soups, or as broth.

Millet—A nutritious grain, easy to digest and quick to cook.

Milk (non-dairy)—Made from rice, soy, almond, or oats. Check your local health-food store for a variety of choices. A healthy substitute for high fat animal products.

Mock coffee—coffee substitute, tastes similar without caffeine, usually made from roasted grains.

Mock turkey—Soy product and healthier substitute for turkey.

Nori—Seaweed sheets used for sushi rolls, you can make avocado rolls without fish.

Nuts and seeds—Buy whole, raw, unprocessed nuts and seeds, which contain healthy fat and building proteins. Try a variety such as sunflower seeds, sesame seeds, flaxseeds, pumpkin seeds, almonds, cashews, pecans, walnuts, filberts, pistachios, brazil nuts, and pine nuts.

Pizza (vegetarian and vegan)—Made on whole-grain crust with healthy toppings, found in the freezer of your heath-food store.

Pero—A coffee substitute, no caffeine, yet tastes similar to coffee, made from roasted grains.

Rice milk—Nondairy milk made from brown rice.

Rice syrup—A healthy sweetener to use in pastries and desserts.

Salt—Earth salt is an unhealthy product. Try using dulse and kelp in shakers, or substitute small amounts of sea salt. Best is to use liquid aminos, see this section.

Soy milk—Nondairy milk made from soybeans.

Sprouts—Young sprouts of edible plants such as alfalfa, sunflower, buckwheat, clover, mung bean, and radish.

Succanat—A healthy, unheated, organically grown, natural granular sugar.

Sugar—Avoid sugar and fructose and all products which contain them, then replace these depleted foods in moderation with Succanat.

Tabouli—A grain salad made from bulgur wheat, comes premade or in packages.

Tahini—Sesame seeds ground into a paste, like peanut butter, high in calcium and protein (choose raw, not roasted).

Tofu—A cheeselike product made from soybeans. Has no animal fat or cholesterol. Use tofu in soups, on sandwiches, or in salads.

Tofu dogs—Healthy substitute for hot dogs, made from soybeans. Save an animal and improve your health at the same time.

Tofu scrambler— Healthy substitute for eggs. A soy product looks and tastes like eggs.

Veggi burger—A burger patty made without meat from grains, nuts, or beans.

Wheat grass juice—Juice of the grass grown from sprouted wheat, considered to be one of the most nutritious foods yet discovered. Buy this juice fresh-squeezed at your health-food store, or purchase a wheat grass juicer and make it yourself.

Whole grain bread—Bread made with the whole grain, no bleached flours, and all natural ingredients.

Yogurt (nondairy)—Yogurt made from soybeans or rice, comes in many fruit flavors.

Young coconut—A coconut in the early stages, contains the best water on the planet, meat is soft and very nutritious.

7-Day Balanced Meal Plan

Before you sit down to your first delicious meal on my diet, you need to remember a few general principles. Review this chapter and pick a level of eating assistance which best supports your transitional needs. Then select a meal from each list by choosing the level that matches your current eating habits. Work within that level while striving for improvement. Gradually move toward the higher-level diets, but at the same time move at your own pace. Don't be afraid to sample meals from other levels. Set yourself a goal, and don't lose sight of it until you have achieved it. If you cannot stick to your diet, stop the program, wait a few days, or weeks, then try again.

All items in the menu below with the asterisk (*) next to them can be found in your local health-food store or your grocer's natural food section.

For proper digestion, all beverages should be consumed 30 minutes prior to eating the meal.

BREAKFAST

LEVEL I	DRINKS	BREAKFAST
	6 oz hot carob drink or mock coffee	2-strips Fakin' Bacon* I cup Tofu Scrambler* I piece whole-grain toast I tbsp natural jam

LEVEL 2	DRINKS	BREAKFAST
	6 oz herb tea w/ tbsp honey and ½ lemon, juiced	I cup steamed whole grain ½ banana *and* 3 oz natural maple syrup

LEVEL 3	DRINKS	BREAKFAST
	10 oz fresh-squeezed apple-celery juice	*Protein Smoothie* 10 oz apple juice, blended w/ I tbsp almonds and ½ banana

LEVEL 4	DRINKS	BREAKFAST
	8 oz fresh-squeezed orange juice w/dash of cayenne pepper diluted 30% with warm filtered water	I peach w/ 4 soaked dried figs and 2 oz nuts

LUNCH (DAY I)

LEVEL I	DRINKS	LUNCH
	8 oz herb tea w/ lemon and honey	*Sandy's Tofu Sandwich* 3 oz tofu w/lettuce, torn, and sprouts 2 slices whole-grain sprout bread

LEVEL 2	DRINKS	LUNCH
	8 oz fresh-squeezed carrot, parsley, apple juice	*Heavenly Veggi Burger* 3 oz patty w/lettuce,

tomato, & alfalfa
sprouts served on 1 whole-
grain sprouted bun

LEVEL 3	DRINKS	LUNCH
	8 oz fresh-squeezed apple, celery, cucumber juice	*California-Style Avocado Sandwich* ½ sliced avocado w/sprouts, spinach, and sun-dried tomato 2 slices whole-grain sprouted bread 2 carrot sticks

LEVEL 4	DRINKS	LUNCH
	8 oz fresh-squeezed parsley, kale, spinach, celery, apple juice	2 cups sprout salad w/ colorful garnish ½ cup guacamole salad 1 cracker—Onion Grain Crisp

DINNER (DAY 1)

LEVEL 1	DRINKS	DINNER
	8 oz fresh-squeezed carrot, celery juice	1½ cup millet grain w/steamed vegetables 2 cups favorite salad 2 slices whole-grain cinnamon Manna bread*

LEVEL 2	DRINKS:	LEVEL 2 DINNER
	8 oz fresh-squeezed carrot, celery juice	1 cup steamed brown rice ½ cup steamed carrots/green beans 1 cup salad of apple, walnut, celery, on bed of greens, w/ 2 oz dressing 1 whole-grain dinner roll

LEVEL 3	DRINKS	DINNER
	10 oz fresh-squeezed carrot, celery, beet juice	1 large tomato, filled w/ 3 oz tofu salad, placed on 1 cup bed of salad greens 1 orange sliced around salad

LEVEL 4	DRINKS	DINNER
	Wheat grass cocktail: 2 oz wheat grass juice 8 oz pineapple juice	4 oz guacamole, placed in ½ avocado shell 2 celery sticks stuffed with 3 oz almond butter*

DAY 2

BREAKFAST (DAY 2)

LEVEL 1	DRINKS	BREAKFAST
	8 oz Pero coffee substitute sweetened with raw honey	1 cup low-fat granola with ½ cup warm rice milk ½ banana and 2 oz raisins

LEVEL 2	DRINKS	BREAKFAST
	8 oz warm apple cider w/ ginger & lemon	1 cup hot whole-grain cereal w/ 4 soaked dried apricots

LEVEL 3	DRINKS	BREAKFAST
	10 oz fresh-squeezed carrot, apple juice	1 blended banana served over 3 fresh figs or 1 sliced apple 1 slice sprouted Manna bread* w/ 2 tbsp almond butter*

LEVEL 4	DRINKS	BREAKFAST
	10 oz fresh-squeezed apple, ginger, kale, celery juice	1 papaya, sliced 3 oz Brazil nuts

LUNCH (DAY 2)

LEVEL I	DRINKS	LUNCH
	8 oz cashew milk w/ cinnamon	*Brown Rice Stuffed Pepper* ½ cup brown rice ⅓ cup steamed vegetables ½ cup rice pudding (dessert)

LEVEL 2	DRINKS	LUNCH
	12 oz fresh-squeezed carrot, spinach juice	2 leaves stuffed spinach rolls 3 oz sun-dried tomato hummus w/ 1½ cup salad greens w/ ½ tomato cut into wedges

LEVEL 3	DRINKS	LUNCH
	10 oz fresh-squeezed cucumber, lettuce juice w/cayenne	2 vegetarian sushi rolls made w/ ⅓ cup brown rice/ avocado filling ½ cup carrot raisin salad ½ orange, juiced 4 tbsp raisins soaked in orange juice

LEVEL 4	DRINKS	LUNCH
	16 oz fresh-squeezed carrot shake w/cashew and spirulina	2 cups mixed green salad w/ dressing 1 cup OJ/blended w/ ½ cup cashews 2 sticks celery stuffed with 3 oz almond butter*

DINNER (DAY 2)

LEVEL I	DRINKS	DINNER
	10 oz fresh-squeezed carrot, lettuce juice	2 cups whole-wheat spaghetti w/ 1 cup mixed green salad

LEVEL 1	DRINKS	DINNER
		1 piece whole-grain garlic bread
		1 oz olive oil

LEVEL 2	DRINKS	DINNER
	10 oz fresh-squeezed carrot, kale juice	1 baked potato stuffed w/ ½ cup guacamole
		1 cup sprout salad
		2 oz dressing

LEVEL 3	DRINKS	DINNER
	8 oz fresh-made almond nut milk	1 cup cooked millet w/ ½ cup steamed vegetables
	1 whole-grain muffin	2 cups spinach salad
		2 oz dressing

LEVEL 4	DRINKS	DINNER
	10 oz fresh-squeezed pineapple green drink- pineapple, celery, parsley, romaine juice	2 cups kale cucumber and tomato salad
		3 oz almond butter rolled in 2 leaves lettuce w/dash liquid amino*
		1 radish sliced for garnish

DAY 3

BREAKFAST (DAY 3)

LEVEL 1	DRINKS	BREAKFAST
	10 oz fresh apple juice w/ginger and ½ lemon, juiced	2 cups steamed rice w/ cinnamon
		2 tbsp honey and 2 oz raisins

LEVEL 2	DRINKS	BREAKFAST
	10 oz fresh-squeezed cucumber, kale juice for the guru on the run	10 oz carrot juice blended w/ ⅓ cup cashews and
		½ frozen, peeled banana
		1 apple bran muffin

LEVEL 3	DRINKS	BREAKFAST
	Citrus punch:	I apple blended w/
	4 oz fresh-made orange juice	⅓ cup raw sunflower seeds
	4 oz grapefruit juice	and I banana
	½ lemon, juiced	

LEVEL 4	DRINKS	BREAKFAST
	I tbsp flaxseeds, blended w/	I fresh peach, apple, or
	2 cups fresh pineapple and	orange
	I cup fresh raw kale and	Slice and enjoy nature's
	I banana	sweetness

LUNCH (DAY 3)

LEVEL I	DRINKS:	LUNCH
	Blueberry Smoothie-blend:	I cup hot vegetarian soup
	10 oz fresh-squeezed orange juice	I½ cup green salad
	½ cup blueberries	2 oz dressing
	½ banana	I 100% sprouted roll
	I tsp bee pollen	

LEVEL 2	DRINKS	LUNCH
	10 oz fresh-squeezed	I cup apple-walnut salad
	tomato, celery juice w/	served on
	dash of liquid amino	I½ cup salad greens w/
		I slice Manna bread*

LEVEL 3	DRINKS	LUNCH
	4 oz almond milk, mixed w/	I cup cream of carrot soup
	4 oz carrot juice	(nondairy)
		I slice Manna bread,
		garnished with
		4 pieces raw broccoli and
		⅓ tomato sliced

LEVEL 4	DRINKS	LUNCH
	10 oz fresh-squeezed	2 cups Yogi Sprout Salad
	chard, celery, and carrot juice	w/ ½ sliced avocado and

LEVEL 4	DRINKS	LUNCH
	Dash of cayenne pepper	dash of granular kelp,* garnish w/¹⁄₃ grated beet

DINNER (DAY 3)

LEVEL 1	DRINKS	DINNER
	8 oz hot peppermint tea 1 tsp honey few drops lemon juice	1¹⁄₂ cup cooked barley w/ ¹⁄₂ steamed veggies 1 piece whole-grain rye bread w/1 cup salad greens

LEVEL 2	DRINKS	DINNER
	10 oz fresh-squeezed celery, parsley, pineapple juice	Tabouli Salad: 1¹⁄₂ cup bulgur wheat, 1 slice millet rice Manna bread, on 1 kale leaf, w/ 2 orange slices garnish

LEVEL 3	DRINKS	DINNER
	10 oz fresh-squeezed apple, celery, romaine lettuce juice	1 baked yam 1 cup steamed broccoli and carrots Sauce: 2 oz olive oil and 1 oz raw cider vinegar

LEVEL 4	DRINKS	DINNER
	10 oz carrot green drink: 5 oz carrot, 5 oz lettuce, spinach, and celery juice	1 apple blended w/ ¹⁄₂ banana 1 tbsp flaxseeds and 2 leaves kale 4 oz springwater

DAY 4

BREAKFAST (DAY 4)

LEVEL 1	DRINKS	BREAKFAST
	Braggs Apple Cider Cocktail:	2 slices Manna bread*
	8oz water	(date-cinnamon)
	2 tbsp raw apple cider vinegar w/	3 oz almond butter and
	1 tbsp honey	1 tbsp honey

LEVEL 2	DRINKS	BREAKFAST
	5 oz fresh-squeezed orange juice mixed w/	1 mango blended w/
	5 oz carrot juice	½ banana, serve over
		½ sliced apple

LEVEL 3	DRINKS	BREAKFAST
	12 oz watermelon juiced w/	½ cantaloupe peeled and
	rind and red meat	sliced

LEVEL 4	DRINKS	BREAKFAST
	5 oz celery, cucumber, and chard juice	1 apple w/
	mixed w/ water of young coconut	3 oz raw macadamia nuts

LUNCH (DAY 4)

LEVEL 1	DRINKS	LUNCH
	8 oz peppermint tea	1 cup vegetarian lentil soup
	1 slice lemon &	1 whole-grain pita pocket
	1 tbsp honey	bread, w/ 4 oz hummus
		2 carrot sticks for garnish

LEVEL 2	DRINKS	LUNCH
	10 oz carrot, celery,	1 stuffed tomato w/
	beet, apple juice	3 oz mock egg salad*
		served on
		1 cup salad greens
		½ kiwi, sliced, for garnish

LEVEL 3	DRINKS	LUNCH
	Berry smoothie:	$1\frac{1}{2}$ cup fruit salad
	4 strawberries	with papaya and mango
	$\frac{1}{2}$ cup blackberries	slices, sprinkled w/
	$\frac{1}{3}$ cup raspberries, blended w/	2 oz sunflower seeds
	8 oz fresh-squeezed orange juice	For dressing:
		Blend $\frac{1}{2}$ banana w/
		$\frac{1}{2}$ tsp honey

LEVEL 4	DRINKS	LUNCH
	10 oz fresh-squeezed (4-seas juice)-	4 soaked figs w/
	chard, celery, carrot, cucumber juice with	3 oz filberts, served on
	dash cayenne pepper	1 purple cabbage leaf

DINNER (DAY 4)

LEVEL 1	DRINKS	DINNER
	1 tomato blended w/	2 dolmas stuffed grape leaves*
	$\frac{1}{2}$ cup spinach	w/3 oz brown-rice filling
	$\frac{1}{2}$ cup springwater	$1\frac{1}{2}$ cup vegetable salad w/
	w/dash cayenne and	1 oz dressing and
	liquid amino to taste	1 slice Manna bread*

LEVEL 2	DRINKS	DINNER
	8 oz peppermint herb Tea	Vegetarian pizza* (nondairy)
	1 tbsp honey	10 oz slice
	1 slice lemon	1 slice whole-grain garlic
		bread
		2 cups salad greens
		2 oz dressing

LEVEL 3	DRINKS	DINNER
	10 oz water from young coconut	$\frac{1}{2}$ cup steamed cauliflower,
		with $3\frac{1}{4}$ cup steamed
		asparagus
		Sauce for vegetables:
		1 orange, juiced, blended
		w/ $\frac{1}{3}$ cup cashews

LEVEL 4	DRINKS	DINNER
	8 oz carrot mixed w/	4 vegetable sushi
	1 oz wheat grass	(California rolls)
		½ cup brown rice
		½ avocado sliced

DAY 5

BREAKFAST (DAY 5)

LEVEL 1	DRINKS	BREAKFAST
	10 oz soy milk, blended w/	1 cup sliced banana
	1 peeled frozen banana	3 oz soaked raisins
		1 slice toasted Manna
		bread* w/
		3 oz almond butter*

LEVEL 2	DRINKS	BREAKFAST
	10 oz warm apple cider, w/	2 cups fruit salad w/
	lemon and ginger to taste	3 oz nuts
		6 oz nondairy yogurt

LEVEL 3	DRINKS	BREAKFAST
	Marathon smoothie:	1 slice sprouted Manna
	3 cups apple juice, blended w/	bread*
	1 banana, peeled and frozen	(millet rice style) w/
	2 tbsp almond butter	3 oz cashew butter and
		1 oz honey

LEVEL 4	DRINKS	BREAKFAST
	10 oz orange juice blended w/	4 soaked brown figs, served
	½ mango and 1 tsp spirulina	w/ 1 banana, sliced, and
		3 oz Brazil nuts

LUNCH (DAY 5)

LEVEL 1	DRINKS	LUNCH
	Mix:	
	8 oz carrot juice	I cup split-pea soup
	2 oz beet juice	2 celery sticks w/
	2 oz apple juice	4 oz guacamole

LEVEL 2	DRINKS	LUNCH:
	8 oz orange, grapefruit juice	I cup creamy potato soup
		2 cups salad greens w/
		$\frac{1}{2}$ tomato, sliced
		I whole-grain cracker

LEVEL 3	DRINKS	LUNCH:
	10 oz apple, celery juice	2 vegetarian sushi roll made
		w/ 3 oz brown rice
		$\frac{1}{2}$ avocado
		$\frac{1}{3}$ tomato sliced into wedges
		on fresh romaine w/ orange
		slices

LEVEL 4	DRINKS	LUNCH:
	10 oz apple juice blended w/	2 cups sprout salad w/
	I tbsp sesame seeds and	3 oz sacred pine nut/
	I tbsp flaxseeds	mango sauce
	I banana	(Blend $\frac{1}{2}$ mango with $\frac{1}{3}$ cup
		pine nuts)

DINNER (DAY 5)

LEVEL 1	DRINKS	DINNER:
	Nut milk	I cup spinach salad w/
	$\frac{1}{3}$ cup sunflower seeds blended w/	$\frac{1}{3}$ sliced tomato and
	10 oz hot water and	3 oz pine nuts, served w/
	$\frac{1}{2}$ banana	I cup steamed yellow squash
		Dessert: I mango blended
		w/ $\frac{1}{2}$ avocado

LEVEL 2	DRINKS	DINNER:
	10 oz cucumber, carrot, apple juice	I cup tabouli salad* 2 leaves romaine lettuce I cup cream of squash soup

LEVEL 3	DRINKS	DINNER:
	10 oz carrot, coconut, parsley juice	I stuffed potato w/ 3 oz tofu salad* I½ cup salad greens 3 oz dressing Dressing:: ½ lemon, juiced w/ 2 oz sesame tahini*

LEVEL 4	DRINKS	DINNER:
	10 oz carrot juice, blended w/ ½ avocado 2 leaves kale	I cup (nondairy) cream of broccoli soup 2 cups kale and macadamia nut salad ⅓ red bell pepper sliced to garnish

DAY 6

LEVEL I	DRINKS	BREAKFAST
	10 oz carrot, apple juice with ginger	Oatmeal w/ ½ banana, 3 oz raisins and I tbsp honey

LEVEL 2	DRINKS	BREAKFAST
	12 oz kiwi, apple smoothie 8 oz apple juice, blended w/ 2 kiwi I banana, peeled and frozen	6 soaked dried apricots w/ 3 oz almonds and 2 fresh dates stuffed w/ 2 oz cashew nut butter*

LEVEL 3	DRINKS	BREAKFAST
	10 oz carrot, orange, parsley juice	1 whole grapefruit

LEVEL 4	DRINKS	BREAKFAST
	2 oz wheat grass juice	1 Papaya, blended w/
	Optional: dilute w/	3 leaves kale, and handful of
	5 oz distilled water	parsley

LUNCH (DAY 6)

LEVEL 1	DRINKS	LUNCH:
	10 oz lettuce, cucumber,	1 stuffed tomato, filled w/
	and pineapple juice	3 oz tabouli salad, served on
		1½ cup salad greens

LEVEL 2	DRINKS	LUNCH:
	Strawberry Smoothie:	2 dolmas*
	10 oz orange juice, blended w/	½ cup brown rice in grape
	1 peeled and frozen banana	leaves
		2 cups salad greens, garnish
		w/ ⅓ sliced yellow squash
		2 oz dressing

LEVEL 3	DRINKS	LUNCH:
	2 oz wheat grass juice w/	2 cups kale salad w/
	4 oz carrot juice chaser	2 oz Italian dressing
		1 slice Manna bread*

LEVEL 4	DRINKS	LUNCH:
	10 oz watermelon,	1 apple blended w/
	cantaloupe juice	2 leaves chard
		⅓ cup sunflower sprouts*

DINNER (DAY 6)

LEVEL 1	DRINKS	DINNER:
	10 oz carrot, celery juice	1 cup brown rice w/
		½ cup steamed broccoli

		½ cup salad greens, w/
		2 oz dressing

LEVEL 2	DRINKS	DINNER:
	10 oz cucumber, carrot, and apple juice	I cup cooked barley w/ ½ cup steamed carrots and spinach I cup carrot-raisin salad

LEVEL 3	DRINKS	DINNER:
	8 oz alfalfa mint tea	I cup Quinoa,* w/ ½ cup steamed green beans I ½ cup mixed green salad 2 oz dressing

LEVEL 4	DRINKS	DINNER:
	5 oz kale, parsley, sunflower sprout, celery, cucumber juice, mixed w/ 5 oz bottled water	2 cups sprout salad w/ ½ sliced avocado, dash of dulse* ½ lemon, juiced garnish w/ ½ orange, sliced

DAY 7 ~ BODY CLEANSING AND DETOXIFICATION

BREAKFAST (DAY 7)

Strive to relax and take it easy on the cleansing day. If possible, avoid any excessive stress and keep your physical activity to a moderate level.

For proper digestion, all beverages should be consumed 30 minutes prior to eating the meal.

LEVEL I	DRINKS:	BREAKFAST:
	8 oz warm bottled water mixed w/ ½ lemon, juiced I tbsp honey	2 apples

LEVEL 2	DRINKS:	BREAKFAST:
	8 oz warm bottled water mixed w/ ½ lemon, juiced I tbsp honey	I apple

LEVEL 3	DRINKS:	BREAKFAST:
	8 oz warm bottled water mixed w/ ½ lemon, juiced I tbsp honey	5 oz cucumber, kale, apple juice, mixed w/ 5 oz bottled water

LEVEL 4	DRINKS:	BREAKFAST:
	8 oz warm bottled water mixed w/ ½ lemon, juiced I tbsp honey	2 oz wheat grass mixed w/ 8 oz water

LUNCH (DAY 7) ~ BODY DETOXIFICATION—CLEANSING

LEVEL I	DRINKS:	LUNCH:
	10 oz fresh-squeezed celery, carrot, parsley	2 cups salad greens w/ ½ avocado sliced ½ lemon squeezed on salad

LEVEL 2	DRINKS:	LUNCH:
	10 oz fresh-squeezed celery, carrot, parsley	2 cups salad greens w/ ½ avocado sliced ½ lemon squeezed on salad

LEVEL 3	DRINKS:	LUNCH:
	8 oz warm bottled water mixed w/ ½ lemon, juiced I tbsp honey	5 oz cucumber, kale, apple juice, mixed w/ 5 oz bottled water

LEVEL 4	DRINKS:	LUNCH:
	8 oz warm bottled water mixed w/ ½ lemon, juiced I tbsp honey	2 oz wheat grass mixed w/ 8 oz water

LEVEL 1	DRINKS:		DINNER:
	8 oz peppermint tea		16 oz fresh-squeezed carrot,
	$\frac{1}{2}$ lemon, juiced		celery juice
	1 tbsp honey		
LEVEL 2	DRINKS:	LEVEL 2	DINNER:
	8 oz warm bottled water mixed w/		10 oz fresh-squeezed celery,
	$\frac{1}{2}$ lemon, juiced		carrot, parsley
	1 tbsp honey		
LEVEL 3	DRINKS:	LEVEL 3	DINNER:
	8 oz warm bottled water mixed w/		5 oz cucumber, kale, apple
	$\frac{1}{2}$ lemon, juiced		juice, mixed w/
	1 tbsp honey		5 oz bottled water
LEVEL 4	DRINKS:	LEVEL 4	DINNER:
	8 oz warm bottled water mixed w/		2 oz wheat grass mixed w/
	$\frac{1}{2}$ lemon, juiced		8 oz water
	1 tbsp honey		

At the end of the cleansing day, do some deep breathing, very light yoga exercise, and get to bed early.

CROSS-TRAINING
WITH A YOGIC
ATTITUDE

To the heavens lift weights
Such gravity you must fight
Then run like wild deer
Into the night

In order to be healthy you need to exercise on a regular basis. If you do not exercise, you will not achieve your full potential and your health will truly suffer. Yoga in itself can create a good amount of fitness, especially if you cross-train with hard and soft techniques of practice. But you will find that there are times when you need a different sort of workout to balance your yoga practice. When you combine yoga with other exercise, you will touch every avenue of your fitness spectrum in a positive way. What's more, your yoga practice will improve from the increase of other physical activity. If you gradually incorporate other physical activities into your exercise program using a yogic attitude, your physical and mental health will be greatly enhanced.

YOUR MIND-BODY CONNECTION FOR GREATER FITNESS

You can use your yoga training to assist you in all other exercise. Probably the most important element of a yogic attitude in terms of other physical activities is developing the mind-body connection. In all phases of yoga we are taught to seek this connection: to live in the moment and approach life with a holistic viewpoint. When you participate in any physical activity, let each movement be sacred and in harmony with your mind. It does not matter whether you are a baseball player, dancer, surfer, or simply going for a brisk walk.

While you can certainly exercise your body without having a complete mind-body connection, if you can focus on your mind while you work your body, your fitness will greatly improve. The following is a four-step plan for enhancing your mind-body connection during traditional physical fitness:

Visualize success and your body will follow. Whenever you are working out or playing sports, try to keep a positive uplifting attitude and visualize yourself doing well. This creative visualization will plant seeds of success in your mind and actually assist you to a better physical workout. Many professional athletes visualize success before they walk onto the playing field. For example, if you were about to pole vault over a very high bar, you would have much better success by visualizing yourself clearing the jump. The same holds true for any physical activity: you can create a positive visualization of your success before you actually put this into action.

Embrace yoga breathing throughout your exercise. Breathing is absolutely essential in any physical or mental task. Before any physical activity, sit quiety for about five minutes and practice slow, deep yogic breathing, completely filling your lungs on inhalations and completely emptying your lungs on exhalations. Strive to breathe through your nose. Calm and relax your mind as you embrace energy on inhalations and relaxation on exhalations.

During exercise, incorporate conscious deep breathing: this will give you more energy and enhance your overall activity. Concious breathing will also lesson the chance of lactic acid buildup in your muscles and allow your muscles a greater chance of recovery after exercise. As you move into your physical activity, you can continue your breathing techniques with some modifications. If you are engaging in light to moderate aerobic exercise, you can practice conscious breathing through your nose, as you do in your yoga breathing techniques. With moderate to heavy aerobic exercise, you will have to make a conscious effort to embrace a continuous and powerful flow of inhalations and exhalations through both your nose and mouth.

Controlling Your Thoughts. During any sort of exercise, it is important to control your mind, to concentrate and focus your every thought on all the details of your body movement and breathing. Sense withdrawal will help you block out distractions and stay focused. Discard outward distractions and focus your thoughts onto your muscles, body movement, and breathing related to your present physical activity. You can allow your mind the freedom to wander for 30 minutes before and again 30 minutes after exercise. It is an easy technique; just drain your random thoughts and relax your focus.

Seeking the Art of Moving Meditation

No matter what sort of exercise you do, remember to maintain an element of spirituality, stay focused on what you are doing, and ultimately embrace a full mind-body connection. The ultimate in any physical activity is to achieve a moving meditation, with a full mind-body connection in a relaxed yet focused manor. You no longer have to push the mind and body into action; this comes naturally as the energy of body and mind merge as one, connecting with the natural flow in the universe. Visualize yourself as a spectator viewing your own activity from the distance in a calm, relaxed state of mind. Be aware of all things, sounds, smells, and actions around you, yet stay focused on your own activity. Allow the energy of your positive thoughts to run free and your body will follow with effortless grace and precision.

Make Your Physical Journey Fun

It has been proven many times over that a lighthearted approach to any physical activity will assist in achieving a successful outcome. A sense of humor is a wonderful base for a true *yogi* or *yogini* who remembers that yoga is noncompetitive and other competition is not ego, simply fun. Winning or losing in competitive sports should both be taken with a lighthearted attitude. Be happy, enjoy your fitness activity, and if this involves others, then welcome their presence and become one with the moment. The journey is everything; so you might as well make it fun.

Using Yoga to Prevent Injury

Aside from experiencing a real feeling of joy, a mind-body connection will also help prevent unnecessary injuries. For example, pulled muscles, twisted knees, and sprained ankles are all caused by fatigue and a break in your mental concentration. Almost everyone who has ever tried running, jogging, or hiking has experienced a sprained ankle at one time or another. This is a classic example of the lack of mind-body connection. If you are focused, aware, and in-tune with your every movement, then a sprained ankle is highly unlikely.

CROSS-TRAINING WITH YOGA

When I first started practicing yoga, I gradually eliminated most other physical activities for a period of about three years. At that time I thought other exercise would cause injuries and I was convinced that the more yoga the better, thinking that other exercise would only get in the way of progress. During this three-year period, I had a host of different injuries, affecting my knees, back, ankles, and wrist. Much to my amazement, it was the lack of balance in exercise which caused the injuries. Too much yoga actually caused an unbalanced physical structure.

While taking part in excessive yoga I had stretched and lengthened all my muscles and joints too much without a balanced strengthening regimen. Aside from physical injuries, I had developed a lethargic attitude from too much yoga, a symptom I now call "yoga drunk." I decided to do an experiment. For about three weeks, I greatly cut back my daily yoga practice, quit doing Lotus Posture and several other extreme postures which involved intense stretching of muscles and joints, and then I starting walking up stairs, hiking hills, riding my bike, and doing abdominal work. After only three weeks, mentally I was full of energy and physically all my injuries were gone. I had created a necessary balance.

In time I gradually added all my yoga postures back into my regular yoga practice routine, along with many other physical activities and all my injuries have totally disappeared. The lesson was fairly clear: if you only do traditional exercise, you will have injuries, stress, tight muscles, and a nonholistic whole body workout, never reaching that blissful plateau or true relaxation. If you just practice yoga alone, as wonderful as it is, you may suffer from becoming overstretched, and lack a hard aerobic activity. The solution is to use yoga as your base, then incorporate other traditional physical and mental activities into a cross-training program.

There is an endless list of physical activities and exercises that complement yoga practice. Perhaps you have some favorites of your own. By incorporating some other moderate additional physical activity into your overall routine, your yoga and overall health will greatly benefit.

You can generally divide all exercise into three categories: aerobic exercise, muscle resistance exercise, and stretching. Some forms of exercise incorporate more than one of these categories, although I will list these individual exercises in their main area of benefit.

AEROBIC EXERCISE

Your very life depends on a strong heart and healthy lungs. This type of exercise involves targeting the strengthening of your heart and lungs. Any exercise which involves continuous sustained physical workouts that cause you to do deep breathing, and elevates your heart to its maximum safe level, is considered to be an aerobic workout. In order to enhance your overall health, strive to practice aerobics for a minimum of 15 to 20 minutes, three to four times a week. With aerobic exercise it is prescribed to elevate your heart rate up to 60 to 75 percent of your maximum rate.

Your Target Heart Zone

Computing the amount of times your heart beats in one minute during exercise is an excellent indicator of the stress on your body. The American College of Sports Medicine defines the recommended zone as 50 to 85 percent of your maximum heart rate. If you do not work out on a regular basis and you are a beginner to exercise, try to stay at the bottom or the 50 percent maximum heartbeat range. If you are in great shape and currently participate in an aerobic program, then you can work in the 70 to 85 percent range of maximum heartbeat.

Finding Your Target Heart Zone

In order to determine your target heart zone, you first have to calculate your maximum heart rate. This formula is an estimate, so your true maximum heart rate could be about 15 beats higher or lower than the results.

Subtract your age from 220, and then multiply this by 50 to 85 percent to find your maximum safe workout zone. For example, if you were 40 years old, you would calculate your maximum target heart zone as in the chart below:

220	220
− 40	− 40
180	180
× .50	× .85
90 beats per minute	153 beats per minute

Measuring Your Heart Rate

One way to determine your heart rate is to take your pulse on your neck or wrist. To test the pulse on your wrist, lightly press your first two fingers at the base of your wrist, on top of the artery that runs by the base of your thumb. For testing your pulse on your neck, place your first two fingers under your chin, just off to one side of center. Count the number of beats for 15 seconds, and then multiply this times 4. If your pulse were beating 10 times in 15 seconds then your heartbeat would be 10 × 4, or 40 beats per minute.

In yoga exercise, some harder forms of yoga embrace a moderate amount of aerobics, yet unless you are very advanced, it is usually not enough to supply you with an ample amount of aerobic workout. If you are an advanced yoga practitioner and do hard-form practice, this activity is still considered mild aerobics as compared to hiking up a steep hill.

Aerobic Cross-Training Ideas

Some of these exercises are mildly aerobic and others are moderate to heavy, yet in moderation, all can serve to enhance your yoga practice, creating a balance in your overall health. Adopt short- and long-term goals to reach your ultimate goal in your chosen activity.

BASEBALL, VOLLEYBALL, RAQUETBALL, TENNIS, AND SOCCER—(Moderate to Heavy Aerobics)
These are all wonderful ways to enjoy a fun, active, and lively game, at the same time enjoying some relaxation. You will find your yoga will give you a much better hand-eye coordination, flexibility to move more freely, and control to make the right moves at the

right time. At the same time these activities will assist in providing a wonderful cross-training exercise for your arms and legs and boosting your aerobics up a notch.

BICYCLING—(Moderate to Heavy Aerobics)
Biking will help strengthen your legs for your standing yoga postures. If you use biking for aerobics, you have to keep a good pace, or ride uphill; if you just glide on the flats, you will not work your cardiovascular system.

WALKING AND HIKING—(Light to Moderate Aerobics)
Walking and hiking are wonderful ways to get a moderate amount of sustained aerobics if you keep a good pace and walk for at least 30 minutes. Walking is great before or after yoga practice, and will assist with warming you up and creating a more vibrant energy flow, as well as helping to avoid injuries. Hiking is also a wonderful way to enjoy your time off and get wonderful aerobic exercise.

JOGGING AND RUNNING—(Moderate to Heavy Aerobics)
Jogging and running are more aerobic than walking and are best done before yoga. Jogging is a preface to running, where you cover less distance in the same amount of time and put out less energy. Unless you are in really good shape, you should stick with jogging. You can work up to jogging by walking with short jogging now and then. You can work up to running by jogging with short interludes of running.

SKIING—(Moderate to Heavy Aerobics)
Skiing is a completely natural form of exercise and excellent ways to release stress and at the same time strengthen your legs. Your yoga will enhance your ability to balance, help to prevent you from getting round shoulders, and stretch out those tight leg muscles and create a necessary balance in overall body alignment. These activities will assist your yoga through strengthening your legs for standing postures, strengthening arms for arm balance postures, and enhanced aerobics which will assist you in the more physical styles of yoga practice.

GOLF—(Light to Moderate Aerobics)
Golf is a wonderful way to release stress and tension, while enjoying a pleasant afternoon on a green lawn. Golf can foster a mind-body connection. Your flexibility, breathing, and relaxed focus in yoga practice will greatly assist you in the physical and mental aspects of

your game. At the same time the relaxed atmosphere of being one with nature can help you find your natural energy connection in yoga practice

SWIMMING—(Moderate Aerobics)
Depending on your level of expertise, this exercise can be aerobic, anaerobic, and relaxing at the same time. Swimming is a great supplement to your yoga practice. Try going for a swim before or after your practice; this is a real treat!

AEROBIC DANCE (Moderate to Heavy Aerobics)
This is a really fun form of aerobic exercise, although be sure to practice your yoga exercise on alternate days with this in order to avoid injury and achieve a balanced spectrum. Be aware of your own limits, drink lots of water, and balance this activity with plenty of yoga.

Muscle Resistance Exercise

Muscle resistance exercise focuses on strengthening, building, and toning the individual muscle groups. Some muscle resistance exercises actually increases the size of your muscles. As you gain more strength with weight-bearing exercise, you will also build bone density, which is very important to your overall health. Evidence supports the fact that weight-bearing exercise helps to prevent osteoporosis, which can often lead to weakness in the bones.

Muscle resistance exercises isolate muscles and work by creating resistance (pushing and pulling). To get results, it is best to practice at least three times a week, for a minimum of 30 minutes each session. In yoga exercise there are many postures which involve pushing your own body weight around, and this in itself is considered muscle resistance exercise. If you choose to get your muscle resistance exercise from yoga, make sure to practice physically challenging postures, hold the postures longer, and try to cover every area of your body. Most often in yoga, no matter how demanding the workout, you are usually pushing your muscles against your own weight, yet lacking the pulling resistance aspect. The pulling is actually the necessary part that creates a balance in the muscle fibers. In order to incorporate pulling into the routine, add chin-ups at the end of your yoga practice, pull weeds in your garden, or incorporate pulling resistance equipment like exercise bands or gym machines into your workout.

Muscle Resistance Cross-Training Ideas

The following muscle resistance exercises can enhance your yoga practice, creating a balance in your overall health. Adopt short- and long-term goals, to reach your own ultimate goal in your chosen activity.

WEIGHT LIFTING

Weight lifting creates muscle resistance through the art of pushing and pulling weights in order to work your muscles. You can use free weights, resistance machines, or if you are a naturalist, lift a boulder in a meadow, or do chin-ups on a tree. If you practice weight lifting, I strongly suggest you do extra yoga to balance the shortening of your muscles. Your weight lifting will assist you in building strength for yoga postures, and your yoga postures will in turn assist you to stretch out those tight muscles along with helping to avoid injuries. If your goal is to tone muscles, use less resistance and do more repetitions, to increase muscle size do more resistance and fewer repetitions.

CALISTHENICS

Calisthenics often crosses over into other categories, such as resistance exercise, aerobics, and stretching. These exercises include sit-ups, push-ups, chip-ups, leg lifts, jumping jacks, and so on. You can start your morning with some light calisthenics to warm up for your yoga exercise: this will complement your practice with strengthening and better aerobics, as well as create a holistic balance. Your regular yoga practice will assist in making calisthenics easier through greater flexibility, more powerful breathing techniques, and enhanced self-confidence. In the Sadhana Yoga program you will receive many of the same benefits as in calisthenics, yet the addition of calisthenics will serve to provide a wider variety and enhance your overall yoga program.

STRETCHING EXERCISES

Stretching refers to the lengthening and loosening of the various muscle groups. Stretching releases tension from your muscles, lengthens the muscle fibers, and increases the range of motion for a muscle or joint. Stretching also increases circulation, is a great way to warm up or cool down, and serves as a wonderful balance for all other physical activities. Your muscles are much more pliable when they are warm, although you should stretch both before and after other exercise for best results. Stretching can also help to prevent post-workout muscle soreness, flexible muscles recover easier than stiff unstretched muscles. Whenever you stretch, take your time and stretch lightly. Respect your limits: trying to stretch too far and too fast can result in pulled muscles and strained tendons.

There are runner's stretches, dance stretches, and many generic fitness stretches, yet none can hold a candle to the stretching within yoga exercise. The stretching in yoga covers every area of your whole body from head to toe. In addition yoga exercise supplies counter-stretches and incorporates synchronized breathing techniques which complement your stretching.

CROSS-TRAINING WORKOUT CHARTS

I have categorized four weekly cross-training workout charts; (Level 1—Beginner), (Level 2—Intermediate), (Level 3—Advanced—A and B). Pick the routine which is most appropriate for your present level of fitness. Remember to always strive to embrace a spiritual element within all avenues of fitness.

BEGINNERS—I consider beginners to be someone new to yoga and fitness, having less than six months' experience, or practicing at a very introductory level. Beginners should take your time; your body will accept gradual change much easier than a radical, sudden change. With overall fitness in mind, what is good for someone else might not be good for you. Let your motives be to exercise for the wonderful feeling it gives you and for the endless health benefits; competition is not always the best avenue for your physical and mental health. There is always a faster gun out there somewhere. Work out with the attitude that everyone who is exercising is a winner; the losers are still sitting on the couch, glued to the TV.

INTERMEDIATE TO ADVANCED—I consider someone to be at the intermediate level when they have at least six months to two years' experience with yoga, and other physical activities practicing at a moderate level. Move toward a gradual change of enhancing your physical activities, don't get extreme and try to do too much too soon, or you may suffer many physical and mental problems. Now and then competition can be fun, when cross-training with nonyoga activities, but don't get obsessed and lose sight of what life is all about. Maintain a yogic attitude; be kind, happy, polite, and generous. Enjoy each and every moment of your day. When you have reached the advanced level, with at least two to four years' experience with yoga, and other cross-training activities, you should practice for personal gain and strive to find a spiritual element in everything you do. Be kind and compassionate, celebrate life and the opportunity to share this experience with your friends.

Below I have outlined three cross-training routines for different levels of practice, mixing yoga with other physical movement. In addition I have listed one routine of cross-training within the spectrum of yoga only. Read the general hints and cautions before you choose a routine.

GENERAL HINTS AND CAUTIONS:

(1) Seek reasonable goals and be patient with yourself.

(2) If possible, try to end your workouts with yoga exercise, or deep relaxation.

(3) Strive to embrace a spiritual element within all your physical activities; embrace the essence of yoga into all areas.

(4) You can add or subtract the time duration within each precribed exercise to fit your own personal needs.

SEVEN-DAY CROSS-TRAINING EXERCISE

(LEVEL 1—BEGINNER)
KARMA YOGA—ACTS OF KINDNESS.

	MONDAY	TUESDAY	WEDNESDAY	THURSDAY	FRIDAY	SATURDAY	SUNDAY
Walk, Jog, or Run	-20- minutes			-30- minutes			
Biking			-20- minutes		-20- minutes		
Calisthenics		-20- minutes		-20- minutes			
General Aerobics						-20- minutes	
Yoga (Hard or Easy)	Easy 40 min		Hard 40 min		Easy 40 min		
Swimming				-20- minutes			
Weight Lifting		-20- minutes				-20- minutes	
Hike or Walk uphill					-30- minutes		
Deep relaxation and Meditation		-30- minutes		-30- minutes		-30- minutes	
Karma Yoga			Karma Yoga 10 minutes				Karma Yoga 10 minutes
Just Relax							All Day

SEVEN-DAY CROSS-TRAINING EXERCISE

(LEVEL 2—INTERMEDIATE)
KARMA YOGA—ACTS OF KINDNESS.

	MONDAY	TUESDAY	WEDNESDAY	THURSDAY	FRIDAY	SATURDAY	SUNDAY
Walk, Jog, or Run	-30- minutes			-30- minutes			
Biking			-30- minutes			-30- minutes	
Calisthenics		-30- minutes		-30- minutes			
General Aerobics			-30- minutes				
Yoga (Hard or Easy)	Easy 75 min.		Hard 60 minutes		Easy 60 min.		
Swimming		-30-min.					
Weight Lifting				-20- minutes		-20- minutes	
Hike or Walk uphill					-60- minutes		
Deep relaxation and Meditation		-30- minutes		-30- minutes		-30- minutes	
Karma Yoga	Karma Yoga 10 minutes		Karma Yoga 10 minutes				Karma Yoga 10 minutes
Just Relax							All Day

SEVEN-DAY CROSS-TRAINING EXERCISE

(LEVEL 3—ADVANCED)
KARMA YOGA—ACTS OF KINDNESS.

	MONDAY	TUESDAY	WEDNESDAY	THURSDAY	FRIDAY	SATURDAY	SUNDAY
Walk, Jog, or Run	-45- minutes			-15- minutes	-45- min.		
Biking			-90- minutes			-60- minutes	
Calisthenics		-45- minutes		-45- minutes		-30- minutes	
General Aerobics			-30- minutes				
Yoga (Hard or Easy)	Easy 90 min.		Hard 90 minutes		Easy 90 min.	Hard 60 min.	
Swimming		-30-min.					
Weight Lifting	-20- minutes			-30- minutes			
Hike or (walk uphill)					-90- minutes		
Deep relaxation and Meditation		-30- minutes		-30- minutes		-30- minutes	
Karma Yoga	Karma Yoga 10 minutes		Karma Yoga 10 minutes		Karma Yoga 10 minutes		Karma Yoga 10 minutes
Just Relax							All Day

SEVEN-DAY CROSS-TRAINING

WITH YOGA ONLY
KARMA YOGA-ACTS OF KINDNESS.

	MONDAY	TUESDAY	WEDNESDAY	THURSDAY	FRIDAY	SATURDAY	SUNDAY
Hard Yoga Workout	45–60 minutes				60–75 minutes		
Easy Yoga Workout		60–90 minutes		45–90 minutes		45–60 minutes	
Partner Adjustments				X			
Outdoor Practice		X					
Day Off Relax			X				X
Endurance Holds						X	
Indoor practice	X			X	X		
Only Relaxation and Meditation			X 30 minutes				X 30 minutes
Karma Yoga			X 10 minutes		X 10 minutes		X 10 minutes

ENDURANCE HOLDS— This refers to holding your yoga posture for two or three times the normal allotted time, or amount of breaths. On this day you would do fewer postures and hold them longer. If necessary practice ⅓ of your routine at a time.

___

PRACTICING
YOGA BEYOND
YOUR MAT

So pursues our existence
The infinite realms of thought
Though ageless secrets
Have always been sought

Once you have mastered the yoga postures and have included meditation, relaxation, and

a balanced diet into your life, you might think that you have done all that yoga has to

offer. In fact, this couldn't be further from the truth. Practicing your yoga postures, you

will feel quite nice. But this is just the beginning. Sadhana Yoga is an avenue to a more

productive and enjoyable life in all ways. Outside of the yoga studio, you can incorporate the physical and mental teachings of yoga into your life, as well as harnessing and utilizing the yoga energy that you have created.

Evaluating Your Energy Source

As you have learned, the practice of yoga connects you with the natural flow of energy throughout the universe. Yoga creates an enormous amount of positive energy. You can choose to store your *prana* on the shelf and let it sit there to collect cobwebs, or put this wonderful and magical gift to work. Sadhana Yoga is especially designed with a holistic approach to help you access your full energy potential. The realization of what you have is the first step along the path to using this energy to assist us in life.

Sadhana Yoga is all about tapping into your full potential, utilizing your body, mind, and spirit in full bloom, unrestricted from distractions of everyday society. If you can use only a minor portion of this energy created from your yoga practice in your daily life, many good things will happen.

PRACTICING YOGA PHILOSOPHY OFF YOUR MAT

When I first started practicing yoga, I was very enthusiastic about being able to touch my toes or do a nice back bend. As my skill level increased, I found myself expanding in all ways. For example, I started reading books that I could not have had the patience to read before. I became interested in learning more about everything from how to make nondairy ice cream to contemplating the energy of the universe. Nature seemed to become a part of my heart, and I saw answers to questions which had not yet been asked. I found that I was changing the way I would approach daily tasks, and I was much more organized and focused. In all ways my self-confidence increased. At first I did not understand what was happening, then one day I knew I was reaping the benefits of yoga beyond my practice mat.

THE SOFT TOUCH OF COMMUNICATION

Mastering the soft touch of communication is the ultimate test of a true *yogi* or *yogini*. You will find that the same idea of "softness is strength" applies to dealing with family, friends, work associates, and others. The highest note in spirituality is communication, you play your note and they play theirs, yet it is not music until they blend. The reality is that simply by communicating, many confrontations can be avoided. The philosophy of

Sadhana Yoga is based on connecting with the natural flow of vital life force energy; this allows the student to greatly enhance their communication skills.

When there is a difference of opinion, it is always much easier to point the finger, blame others, and act with physical and mental anger. In the long run this action will not eliminate the cause, only cover it up, like sweeping the dirt under your carpet. Long-term solutions take a compassionate view of the underlying cause and require a bridge of communication on your part. "Softness is strength" also relates to reaching out your metaphorical hand and making a compassionate effort to calm troubled waters. Good words cost no more than bad and are the most powerful tool at your disposal. Softness also involves the shedding of your ego, forgetting who was right or wrong, and trying to calmly communicate instead to raising your voice or resorting to physical and mental abuse.

Improving Family Life

For many of us, getting along with family is not always as easy as it sounds. Different generations, interests, values, and ethics can make home life a bit rocky from time to time. Fortunately your yoga and *prana* energy can assist you in dealing with family conflicts.

When I was in seventh grade, I began to realize I had a different way of viewing life than my parents. For that matter, I had a different way of viewing life from almost everyone else I knew. I always knew that I was lucky to have wonderful, loving parents. Yet in spite of this, by the time I was seventeen there was a full-blown generation gap between us, and even my sister, who was only two years older than I, seemed to be from another planet.

Many seemingly small issues between parents and children can accumulate and turn into a really big deal. My parents didn't like that I was a vegetarian, or that I chose to wear my hair long with a beard to match. They were very disappointed when I rejected a high-paying corporate oil job and accepted a job in the local health store. To top it all off I started practicing yoga, and let me tell you, yoga was not cool in Texas during the late sixties!.

With a lot of patience, faith in tomorrow, and a lot of work, my parents and I have survived with our relationship still intact. But it wasn't always easy. I learned to take a yogic path to resolve my family issues. I tried to view the world from a position of expansion rather than tunnel vision. This meant that I needed to learn to view things from another's point of view, no matter how abstract it might seem. I also learned to be more patient, and that time itself has a way of healing many problems.

Try out some yogic compassion and understanding, just as you would like to receive from others. The next time you have a confrontation or comfort issue with someone in your family and you get a bit bent out of shape, try taking a nice long walk, or practice a good flowing yoga routine, ending with a wonderful relaxation. Make yourself a shot of wheat grass. Given time, life will seem a bit less nasty afterward, and many answers might become visible, like a beautiful rainbow after a nasty thunderstorm.

Above all, you can always share some of your newfound yoga wisdom through your physical actions. Try to introduce your family to some yoga and deep relaxation. The following routine is developed to be successful with newcomers to yoga for enhancing family relations.

ENHANCED FAMILY YOGA ROUTINE

SEATED POSTURE

Perfect Posture	(see pg. 53)
Yoga breathing	(see pg. 37)

WARM-UPS

Sun Salutation (Soothing Touch I)	(see pg. 66)

or

Cat Stretch Posture (2–10 repetitions)	(see pg. 64)

STANDING POSTURES

Extended Triangle Posture	(see pg. 123)
Sundial Posture	(see pg. 133)
Warrior I Posture	(see pg. 135)
Soft Touch *Vinyasa* (Down)	(see pg. 143)

Staff Posture	(see pg. 87)
Head Knee Posture (2 repetitions)	(see pg. 91)

BACK-BENDING POSTURES

Cobra Posture (2 repetitions)	(see pg. 100)

or

Bow Posture (2 repetitions)	(see pg. 104)
Half Locust Posture	(see pg. 102)

ARM BALANCE POSTURES

Crane Posture (2 repetitions)	(see pg. 118)
Handstand (2 repetitions)	(see pg. 76)

or

Downward Facing Dog Posture (2 repetitions)	(see pg. 113)

INVERTED POSTURES

Shoulder Stand	(see pg. 81)
Bridge Posture (2 repetitions)	(see pg. 84)

RELAXATION POSTURES

Deep Relaxation (5–15 minutes)	(see pg. 140)
Yoga Breathing	(see pg. 37)

Enhancing Relations with Friends

Friends and lovers are priceless gifts; make sure you fully appreciate them. Life is short and moments are precious gems to be valued with the highest esteem. We all have issues of communication with friends, or with lovers; this is just part of living life the best you can. Problems are actually wonderful gifts in disguise, or lessons for you, as the evolution of knowledge continually grows and expands.

A true friend is the one who is there for you at any time, not just when things are going your way. A friend is someone you can confide in no matter what the circumstances might be. We all need friends with whom we can hang out, laugh, talk about life, and reflect on colorful moments in time. Along the yogic path of friendship, you practice unconditional support as long as your effort is focused on generating something positive.

Within the spectrum of friends, never surrender your own true self, or give up what you think is right, sound, and true, just to comply with your perception of peer pressure. As my brother and fellow yoga teacher, David Swenson, once said, "Only dead fish go with the flow!"

I remember vividly in my early years of high school, I was terrified at the thought of trying to be myself. I knew that I was going to have problems being a surfer and an aspiring *yogi* in South Texas. Fortunately, I had a really cool sister who was one of the few people who stood up for me, even when it went against the grain of the masses. My sister Diana once said if your friends couldn't accept you as you are, then they are not really your friends.

The Quality of Friends

When I first started practicing yoga, I was taking a summer surfing vacation in Southern California. Athena, the goddess of the ocean, was my true love. For the chance to ride good waves for just one day, I would gladly quit my job, ditch my girlfriend, sell my car, and hop on a plane to Mexico. Well, during this summer I was fortunate enough to discover a place which had great waves and good yoga teachers. When the waves were not the best, you could find me in the local yoga studio, hanging out with the yoga crowd. When the waves were happening, I would spend all my time at the beach with fellow surfers.

My surfer friends could not understand why I was interested in the weird movement of yoga; after all I was a surfer dude. And my yoga friends gave me a hard time for missing class for weeks on end, when the waves were cranking; after all I was an aspiring *yogi* messing up my alignment. My hippie friends thought it was all way cool, as long as you were totally baked on one thing or another. My straight-edge, conservative friends thought I had totally lost my mind on all accounts.

Yogis and surfers, hippies and straight edgers, they were all my friends and I valued them all equally. In time I found I learned just as much from the negative aspects of my friends as I did the positive aspects. As my yoga progressed, I found common ground with all my friends, I learned to see the world through their eyes and at the same time hold true to my own values. We are all teachers and students. Some of the most unlikely people are the best teachers and they don't even know it. On the other hand some of the ones who took on the air as great teachers, in my opinion, had nothing to offer at all.

Practicing Yoga with Your Friends

No matter who your friends are, or what they do, you can greatly enhance your relationships with them by joining together in the following yoga routine. All minds become one as you share in the feeling of the natural flow of the universe. You can help each other with the magical flow of *asana* within a beautiful nature setting. Your yoga will greatly enhance your friendship, and the collective energy you create can touch many hearts at once.

PRACTICING YOGA WITH FRIENDS

SEATED POSTURES

Perfect Posture	(see pg. 53)
or	
Lotus Posture	(see pg. 55)
Yoga breathing	(see pg. 37)

WARM-UPS

Soft Touch *Vinyasa* I (Upward)	(see pg. 143)
Sun Salutation (Soothing Touch 1)	(see pg. 66)
Sun Salutation (Ultimate Power 2)	(see pg. 71)

Yoga breathing	(see pg. 37)
Deep Relaxation (15 minutes)	(see pg. 140)

YOGIC SPECTRUM OF LOVERS

Yoga will give you self-confidence and help you get in touch with your inner feelings. You cannot fully love or be loved unless you are in touch with your true self. Being in love is a magical emotion: if we can channel this energy into our daily life, we will all be blessed.

In yoga philosophy, there are basically four kinds of love:

(1) **Universal Love**—The love for life and love for all things, which is what peace and compassion is all about. Universal love is in the best interest of all life and the whole human race.

(2) **Energy and Material Love**—The love for an idea, concept, material possession, or specific area or thing. You can love your pet, your job, the idea of swimming in the tropics, or your new car.

(3) **Platonic Individual Love (nonintimate relationship)**—You may have a great love and admiration for someone without the desire to move this friendship into a romantic or physical relationship.

(4) **Intimate Love**— to be involved with someone on an intimate level, much more than friendship. Someone with whom you share your most intimate affection and feelings with.

Intimate Love in a Relationship

Lust and love are two different things. We are all attracted to someone in our life at one time or another. This attraction is often magical, yet love is a deeper well which touches the very soul, creating a harmony of body, mind, and spirit. For a *yogi* or *yogini* to be truly in love, you will have found a lover you find inwardly attractive as well as outwardly attractive. Be patient and let love happen naturally: it is not a business deal or a shopping adventure. Life is always changing; the strongest love can grow out of simple friendship. When the time is right and the universe is ready, your lover will appear.

Communication is of ultimate importance in a relationship. If you are not attentive to this, misunderstandings occur time and again. Try to see life through your lover's heart and eyes, not just through you own personal attraction for their appearance. Be compassionate, understanding, and thoughtful, yet at the same time don't totally surrender your own true self to please another's wishes. Intimate love is all about compromise and communication.

Yoga can greatly help you to enhance all four aspects of love. The path to yoga is a magical journey and if you open your heart and let the *prana* you have created in your yoga practice move into other areas of your life, your love will flourish. All things considered, yoga will enhance your potential to love and to be loved. Try the following yoga routine to enhance your love.

ENHANCING LOVE WITH YOGA

SEATED POSTURES: SIT BACK TO BACK WITH YOUR PARTNER, OR BY YOURSELF

Perfect Posture	(see pg. 53)
or Lotus	(see pg. 55)
Yoga Breathing	(see pg. 37)

WARM-UPS

Cat Stretch Posture (4 repetitions)	(see pg. 64)
Folded Leaf Posture (*massage back of your partner*)	(see pg. 138)
Sun Salutation (Soothing Touch 1) (4 repetitions)	(see pg. 66)
Sun Salutation (Ultimate Power 2) (4 repetitions)	(see pg. 71)
Soft Touch *Vinyasa* I (Downward)	(see pg. 143)

Headstand	(see pg. 76)
Folded Leaf Posture (*massage back of your partner*)	(see pg. 138)
Shoulder Stand	(see pg. 81)
Fish Posture (2 repetitions)	(see pg. 85)

LEG STRETCH POSTURES

Staff Posture	(see pg. 87)
Seated Forward Bend (2 repetitions)	(see pg. 88)
Expanded Foot Posture Variation 5	(See Page 133)

BACK STRETCH POSTURES

Cobra Posture (2 repetitions)	(see pg. 100)
Half Locust Posture	(see pg. 102)
Handstand	(see pg. 120)

Or

Downward Facing Dog Posture (2 repetitions)	(see pg. 113)

ARM BALANCE POSTURES

Scale Posture	(see pg. 116)
Peacock Posture	(see pg 114)

Or

Crane Posture	(see pg. 118)
Soft Touch *Vinyasa* (Upward)	(see pg. 143)

THE WORLD AROUND YOU

In all aspects of your life, the most powerful weapon at your disposal is the ability to love, and the most valuable tool is communication. If words can create negative emotions, or war, then words can prevent or overcome these same outcomes. The solution is very simple; as a yoga student, it is your duty to uphold positive communication, strive to bridge gaps, make compromises, bend in the wind, and hold peace in your heart.

No one student, teacher, spiritual leader, or *guru* has all the answers, yet you have the answer within you. Peace starts within. You can learn abundant, wonderful knowledge from many highly respected people, yet you still must embrace all this knowledge, blending it within your own mind, in order to create the ultimate recipe for life.

All ways are right and one way is wrong. Sunlight is nothing without the darkness, and darkness needs sunlight to highlight its effects. There is a saying: "Cracks within the system allow the light to shine in; therefore, you can see more clearly." Really listen when others speak, feel what is in their heart, and try to see the world through their eyes, just as you would ask them in turn to listen to you.

After many years of practicing yoga I have searched for wisdom in churches and in temples, on Earth and in heaven, with *gurus* and preachers, yet upon completing the cycle I have found the sacred answers and wisdom was always within my own true self. True enlightenment is within you; this you will not find on a deserted tropical island or a mountain paradise. Always remember, along the path of yoga and in life, only hard work builds paradise!

REAPING THE BENEFITS OF HAVING A DAILY PURPOSE

Another important yogic philosophy is to have a daily purpose or passion in life. We all need something special to get us out of bed in the morning. Whatever this daily purpose is, your yoga practice will fuel your interest in a positive way.

Have you ever tossed a pebble into a quiet pond? If not, you should give it a try; this very simple and relaxing act will help to portray your presence on Earth. As you toss a pebble into the quiet pond, the ripples created expand and reach the distant shores. In this life your speaking, writing, and actions create ripples in time for those in future generations who will be in some way affected.

You can send a positive message of preservation, kindness, compassion, and love, or you can send a negative message of destruction, violence, hate, and selfish greed. Everything starts from within: your thoughts are seeds, and if you plant some positive thoughts, these seeds will grow into positive action. Practice yoga and a holistic natural life and you will create harmony within. Tap in to this valuable resource of energy, embracing the power and compassion of *prana* throughout your life. Be aware of your actions, thoughts, and words; this not only effects you and those around you, but in one way or another will touch all those in future generations.

Yoga continues to gain popularity at an alarming rate as our society realizes the precious gifts which are born from this sacred practice. Everyone can benefit from these ancient techniques which act as a stepping-stone to a better way of life and a more enhanced spiritual vision. These gifts within this book are not mine to keep, nor yours, yet this sacred message of timeless energy is to be shared with all, in the stream of life.

The knowledge and information within this book has the ability to affect a great many people in a positive way. I rely on you as the most important medium to carry it out. I hope you have found as I have that Sadhana Yoga is more than just another form of yoga; it's a path to a better way of life, which will touch the hearts and minds of many throughout time.

RESOURCES

YOGA AND PHILOSOPHY BOOKS

Ashtanga: The Practice by David Swenson, David Swenson Productions, 1999.

Essene: Gospel of Peace by Szekely, IBS December, 1981.

Light on Yoga by B. K. S. Iyengar, Shocken Books, January 1966.

Power Yoga for Dummies by Doug Swenson, Hungry Minds, 2001.

Power Yoga by Beryl Bender Birch, Simon and Shuster, 1995.

The Yoga Sutras by Swami Satchidananda, Integral Yoga Publication, 1991.

Yoga/Ernest Wood by Dr. Ernest Wood, Pelican Books, 1959.

HEALTH, DIET, AND NUTRITION BOOKS

Miracle of Fasting by Paul Bragg, Health Science, 1991

Become Younger by N. W. Walker, Norman Walker Publications, September 1995.

Conscious Eating by Gabriel Cousens, M.D., North Atlantic, 2000.

Mucusless Diet Healing System by Arnold Ehret, Ehret Literary, 1994.

Sunfood Diet Success System by David Wolfe, Maul Bros., 2000.

The Hippocrates Diet by Ann Wigmore, Avery, 1984.

The Hunza Trip by Bernard Jensen, Bernard Jensen International, 1990.

MUSICAL SUGGESTIONS FOR MEDITATION

The Harmonic Vibrations of Crystal Singing Bowls by Crystal Voices. This CD is composed of the very unique and relaxing sounds of crystal singing bowls combined with some voice, chimes, and sound of running water. The package includes a guided meditation to clear the chakras, or energy centers, in your body.

Waking the Cobra by Baird Hersey. This CD features nice overtone chanting in which the voice produces a unique higher tone. The slow meditative chanting is perfect for meditation and it also includes pieces to help clear the energy centers of your body. (*www. waking-the-cobra.com*)

Higher Ground by Steven Halpern. This CD provides a slow, mellow, and steady sound that is designed to help you completely relax. (*www.stevenhalpern.com*)

Live on Earth by Krishna Das. If you are new to chanting and want to learn chanting, this is a fun, energetic CD. Kirtan style chanting is done in call and response fashion: the singer sings the words and the crowd then repeats it back. The words and some detailed explanations are included in the sleeve. (*www.krishnadas.com*)

Medicine Power by Oliver Shanti and friends. This is Native American music which has a spiritual message as well as a soothing relaxing melody. Great for meditation or a moving meditation dance. (*www.sattva.com*)

SANSKRIT GLOSSARY

Adho—Downward direction.

Adho Mukha—Downward facing.

Adho Mukha Svanasana—The Downward Facing Dog Posture.

Adho Mukha Vrksasana—The Downward Facing Tree Posture.

Ahimsa—Noninjury, nonviolence, harmlessness.

Ajna—Third eye point, located in the middle of your forehead between your eyes.

Akarna—Near or toward the ear.

Akarna Dhanurasana—The Shooting the Bow Posture.

Ananda—Bliss, which is complete physical and mental paradise.

Anasura—Flowing with grace.

Anga—A limb, or part of your body limbs.

Angustha—The big toe.

Anusara—"Flowing with grace."

Aparigraha—Nongreed, to refrain from hoarding and be free from bonds of materialism.

Ardha—Half.

Ardha Chandrasana—The Half Moon Posture.

Ardha Matsyendrasana—The Half Twist Posture.

Ardha Padamasana—The Half Lotus Posture.

Ardha Salabhasana—The Half Locust Posture.

Asana—A body pose or yoga posture, translates as meaning "position comfortably held."

Ashram—A hermitage; monastery, or sacred temple.

Ashtanga—Eight limbed.

Ashta—Eight.

Asteya—Refrain from stealing and cheating.

Atma—Jnana-Knowledge of the Self.

Atman—The Self, or a term for the enlightened one, self-realized.

Ayurveda—Ancient holistic Indian medical system that places emphasis on the individual's involvement in his or her own well-being.

Baddha—Bound, or caught.

Baddha Padmasana—Bound Lotus.

Bakasana—A crane.

Bala—A child.

Balasana—Child's Posture.

Bandha—A seal or lock. Contraction of internal muscles used to help control *pranic* energy, increase stability in postures and create strength form the core.

Bhagavad Gita—Primary text of Hindu philosophy; contains essential yoga concepts.

Bhakti—Devotion.

Bhuganga—A snake, or a serpent.

Bhujangasana—Cobra Posture.

Brahmacharya—Purity, chastity, non-lust. Relates to the practice of celibacy, or maintaining integrity of intimate relationships. Can also mean purity in thought, word, and action.

Brahman—The Absolute Reality; God.

Buddha—Relates to the Buddha, a man who reached (enlightenment), one who is totally purified from all defilements and who is self-realized.

Chakora—A partridge.

Chakras—Spinning energy wheels in the subtle body, relates to invisible centers of energy within the human system.

Chandra—The moon.

Chatur—Four.

Chaturanga—Four limbed.

Chaturangasana Dandasana—The Four Limbed Staff Posture.

Chela—Disciple, or aspiring yoga student.

Chi—In Chinese philosophy, chi is vital life force energy.

Danda—Staff, or rod.

Dandasana—The Staff Posture.

Dhanu—A bow.

Dhanurasana—The Bow Posture.

Dharana—Concentration, striving to focus all your energy on a particular area of thought.

Dharana—Concentration.

Dharma—Duty; characteristics, righteousness.

Dhyana—Meditation, effortless focus, sustained flow of relaxed thought.

Divya-Drishti—Inner vision, or divine perception.

Dristhi—Point of gaze.

Dwi—Two.

Dwi Pada—Both feet, or both legs.

Eka—Single, one, or alone.

Eka Pada—One foot, or one leg.

Eka Pada Sirsasana—One Leg Behind Head Posture.

Garudasana—Eagle Posture.

Ghee—Natural clarified butter, which has been cooked at low heat.

Gita—Relates to the renowned sacred text *Bhagavad-Gita*.

Guna—A quality born of nature and laws of nature.

Guru—Spiritual teacher, preceptor.

Ha—Syllable meaning the sun, heat, or masculine energy.

Hanumanasasna—The Leg Split Posture (splitting legs front to back).

Hala—A plough.

Halasana—The Plough Posture.

Hasta—Hand.

Hatha Yoga—Yogic system of balancing the body's physical, mental, and spiritual energies.

Ida—The left nerve channel, which corresponds to cooling lunar energy.

Isvara—Lord, God, or ultimate energy.

Jalandhara Bandha—Upper *bandha*, relates to chin lock.

Japa—repetitive prayer, or mantra.

Janu—The knee.

Janu Sirsanana—The Head Knee Posture.

Jiva—Means a living being, the individual Soul.

Jivanmukti—Relates to one who is liberated in this life.

Jnana—Wisdom, or knowledge of the Self.

Jnana Mudra—Traditional yogic hand gesture. The tip of the index finger (representing the individual soul) is brought in contact with the tip of the thumb (representing knowledge of the universe).

Jnana Marga—The path of knowledge.

Kapalabhati—Cleansing breath.

Kapota—A pigeon.

Kapotasana—The Pigeon Posture.

Karma—Your work or action.

Kona—Angle.

Kripal—Compassion or mercy.

Krouncha—A heron.

Kumbaka—Relates to breath retention.

Kundalini—A popular style of yoga practice. The word comes from the root *Kundal*, which indicates the uncoiling of a lock of hair. This symbolizes uncoiling the dormant, sleeping energy located within the individual.

Kurma—A tortoise.

Kurmasana—The Tortoise Posture.

Karna—The ear.

Mantra—A sacred syllable, thought, or word, or set of words sung through repetition with reflection of which one attains a state of meditation.

Manna—A gift from God.

Matsya—Fish.

Matsyasana—Fish Posture.

Matsyendrasana—The Twist Posture.

Maya—Relates to the illusive power of God.

Mayura—A peacock.

Mayurasana—The Peacock Posture.

Mudras—Hand gestures that direct the life current through the body.

Mula Bandha—Root lock, lowest *bandha*, internal sealing or lock. Engaged by contracting or lifting the perineum muscle.

Mukti—Relates to liberation.

Nadis—Invisible energy channels within the body, which serve to carry *prana* energy.

Namaskara—Salute, honoring, or worship.

Namaste—This Hindu salutation says "The divine in me honors the divine in you."

Nava—A boat.

Navasana—The Boat Posture.

Nauli—Abdominal muscle churning, which massages and invigorates internal organs.

Neti—Yogic cleansing techniques to clean the nasal passage.

Nirvana—A state of liberation, or final emancipation.

Niyamas—In the *Yoga Sutras*, Pantanjali defined five *niyamas* or observances relating to inner discipline and responsibility.

Om—The sacred vibration, or monosyllable which symbolizes Brahman.

Pada—Foot.

Padamasana—Full Lotus Posture.

Parivrtta—Revolved, or turned around.

Parivrtta Janu Sirsasana—Twisted Head Knee Posture.

Parivrtta Trikonasana—The Twisted Triangle Posture.

Parivrtta Parsvakonasana—The Twisted Side Flank Angle Posture.

Parsva—Flank, or side.

Pasa—A noose.

Pashasana—Noose Posture.

Paschima—Western, or the back side of your body.

Paschimottanasana—Seated Forward Bend Posture, or western stretch.

Prana—Vital life force energy, the spark of all life.

Pranayama—Rhythmic control of breath used to increase prana and reduce obstructions in the body and mind.

Prasarita—Stretched or spread out.

Prasarita Padottanasana—The Expanded Foot Posture.

Pratyahara—Relates to withdrawal of the senses.

Puraka—Relates to the act of inhalation.

Purva—The east, or the front side of your body.

Purvottanasana—Incline Plane, or Eastern Stretch Posture.

Raja—King: Raja Yoga is mastery over the mind.

Rechaka—Relates to the act of exhalation.

Sadhana—Practice quest, or quest toward mastery.

Salabha—A locust.

Salabhasana—The Locust Posture.

Samadhi—Superconsciousness, self-awareness, a oneness with the universe.

Sanskrit—The ancient language of Hinduism and the Vedas and the classical literary language of India.

Santosa—To embrace contentment within simplicity, and feel tranquility.

Sarva—Whole, or all.

Sarvangasana—The Shoulder Stand Posture.

Sattva—Purity.

Satya—Truthfulness and honesty in all ways.

Saucha—Strive for purity in body, mind or spirit.

Sava—A corpse.

Savasana—The Corpse Posture.

Setu—A bridge.

Setu Bandhasana—The Bridge Posture.

Siddhasana—Perfect Posture.

Simha—Lion.

Simhasana—The Lion Posture.

Sirsa—Your head.

Sirsasana—Headstand Posture.

Sukha—Pleasant, or easy.

Surya—The sun.

Surya-namaskar—Sun Salutation—sequence involving twelve separate but flowing postures.

Svana—A dog.

Svadhyaya—The process of inquiring into your own nature, the nature of your beliefs, and the nature of the world's spiritual journey.

Swami—Title of respect for a spiritual master.

Tada—A mountain.

Tadasana—Mountain Posture.

Tantra—Yogic system that uses the energies of the body, sometimes the sexual energies, to transcend worldly attachments.

Tapas—To work hard and have a burning desire to accomplish something, in order to achieve a positive result.

Tha—Syllable meaning the moon, feminine energy, or cooling.

Tittibha—A flying insect, like a firefly.

Tittibhasana—The Flying Insect Posture.

Tola—A scale.

Tolasana—The Scale Posture.

Tri—Three.

Trikona—A triangle.

Trikonasana—The Triangle Posture.

Uddiyana Bandha—Flying up. It is a core *bandha*, internal sealing or lock.

Ujjayi Breathing—Means victorious breath, yoga sound breathing, achieved by contracting the throat muscles on inhalations and exhalations.

Upavistha—Seated.

Upavistha Konasana—The Seated Angle Pose.

Urdhva—Extended upward, or raised.

Urdhva Dhanurasana—The Upside Down Bow Posture.

Urdhva Mukha Svanasana—Upward Facing Dog Posture.

Utkata—Extraordinary.

Utkatasana—The Powerful Chair Posture.

Uttana—A deliberate, or intense stretch; extended.

Uttanasana—The Standing Forward Bend.

Utthita—Stretched, or extended.

Utthita Hasta Padangusthasana—Sundial Posture.

Ustra—A camel.

Vajra—Thunderbolt.

Vajrasana—Thunderbolt Posture.

Vedas—The highest authority among the Aryans of India.

Vinyasa—The flowing, connecting link between yoga postures.

Vira—A hero, bravery, or warrior.

Virabhadrasana—The Warrior Posture.

Visnu— A deity, entrusted with preservation of the world.

Vrksa—A tree.

Vrksasana—The Tree Posture.

Vrschika— A scorpion.

Vrschikasana—The Scorpion Posture.

Yama—Control.

Yamas—Ethical disciplines for how to treat others.

Yoga—Union, or yoke. Relates to union of physical, mental and spiritual self through the practice of yoga.

Yogi—Male yoga student.

Yogini—Female yoga student.

ABOUT THE AUTHOR

Doug Swenson is an internationally known yoga teacher and rated as one of the best yoga instructors in the country. He began studying yoga in 1967 with Doctor Ernest Wood. In 1972 Doug started teaching yoga classes in colleges and private sessions in his home. More than thirty years later, Doug continues to live the message taught in this book. Doug is the author of several books on yoga and one on diet and nutrition. He teaches Sadhana Yoga workshops all over the world to thousands of students every year.

Doug has been invited to attend the most prestigious yoga conferences, including those sponsored by the *Yoga Journal* and the Omega Institute. At these conferences Doug teaches along with many of yoga's most renowned teachers, including Baron Baptiste, Beryl Bender Birch, Stephen Cope, David Life, Shiva Rea, and Rodney Yee.

Sadhana Yoga—Doug's new style of practice:
for more information for student and teacher certification contact:
Doug Swenson
dougtahoe@hotmail.com
www.sadhanayogachi.com